AF651626

NUTRITION AND DIGESTION

Nutrition and Digestion

J. Christopher

ANMOL PUBLICATIONS PVT. LTD.
NEW DELHI - 110 002 (INDIA)

ANMOL PUBLICATIONS PVT. LTD.
4374/4B, Ansari Road, Daryaganj
New Delhi - 110 002
Ph.: 23261597, 23278000

B.O.: No. 1015, Ist Main Road, BSK IIIrd Stage
IIIrd Phase, IIIrd Block,
Bangalore - 560 085 (India)
Visit us at: www.anmolpublications.com

Nutrition and Digestion

© Reserved

First Published, 2006

ISBN 81-261-2650-7

[Responsibility for the facts stated, opinions expressed, conclusions reached and plagiarism, if any, in this book is entirely that of the Author. The Publishers bear no responsibility for them, whatsoever.]

PRINTED IN INDIA

Published by J.L. Kumar for Anmol Publications Pvt. Ltd., New Delhi - 110 002 and Printed at Mehra Offset Press, Delhi.

Contents

Preface

Physiology is the branch of Biology concerned with the normal functions of living organisms and their parts. An important branch of Science, it is one of the subjects of study of various curricula. From head to toe, every part of body, its structure, functions, formation, safety and security and its proper usage for better results and utilization etc. are some of the core points of discussion in this discipline.

Like anything, animal body also passes through the stages of creation, growth, decay and end. Since change is the basic property of matter, lots of changes occur in the body with the passage of time. Therefore, to keep body fit for a happy life, it needs regular maintenance. This maintenance may be made by taking into account the following points : (i) Systems of Animal Body; (ii) Functions of Animal Body; (iii) Nutrition and Digestion (a must) and (iv) Biochemical Elements.

The present mini-encyclo is an humble endeavour in bringing together the four points at one place. It is not only a book for students and competition aspirants, but also a ready reference for professionals and academics alike.

Any suggestions worth consideration for an enhanced version would be solicited and appreciated.

Editor

1

The Nourishment

Animals need nourishment for three major purposes: (1) to provide the body with energy for performing the various life activities like muscle contraction, movements etc., (2) to maintain the body heat, and (3) to synthesize body substances for growth and repair of the worn out tissues. In animals, the food requirements are met with by the intake of organic compounds of plant or animal origin.

Components of an Adequate Diet : There are 6 major components of the diet : Carbohydrates, Fats, Proteins, Vitamins, Minerals and Water

Of these, carbohydrates, fats and proteins yield energy provide for growth, and maintain tissues subjected to wear and tear. While all 3 major nutrients yield energy to the body: carbohydrates and, to a lesser extent, fats are physiologically the most economical sources. Proteins serve primarily to provide for tissue growth and repairs; but if the caloric intake from other foods is inadequate, they are burned for energy. Vitamins, minerals and water, although they do not yield energy, are essential parts of the chemical mechanisms for the utilization of energy and for the synthesis of various necessary metabolites such as hormones and enzymes. The minerals are also incorporated into the structure of the tissue and, in solution, play an important role in acid-base equilibrium. If the cells of the body are to be able to function efficiently, these nutritional elements must be available to the animal in the correct proportions. A food of this sort, therefore, is often described as the balanced diet.

Carbohydrate Intake

Carbohydrate is the first and most efficient source of energy for vital processes. The principal sources of carbohydrates in foods are :

(i) *glucose* (grape sugar), *fructose* (fruit sugar) and *galactose* [monosaccharides] (ii) *maltose* (malt sugar), *lactose* (milk sugar) and *sucrose* (cane or beet sugar) [disaccharides]. (iii) *Starches, cellulose, glycogen* and *dextrins* [polysaccharides]

It is considered that a minimum of 5 g of carbohydrate per 100 kcal of the total diet is necessary to prevent the development of ketosis, but prevention of the untoward effects of fasting or of high-fat diets will require 50—100 gm of digestible carbohydrates per day.

Functions of Carbohydrates in the Body

(1) *Major Source of Energy* : Almost all animals use carbohydrates as respiratory fuels. In the form of glucose and glycogen, they serve as an important source of energy for vital activities.

(2) *Key-Role in Metabolism* : In the metabolic process of gluconeogenesis, carbohydrate can be supplied from most amino acids as well as from the glycerol moiety of fats.

(3) *Provides Roughage* : Roughage is the undigestable part of the carbohydrate diet, for example, cellulose of fruit, vegetables, salads and wheat-husk. It gives bulk to the diet and, therefore helps to satisfy the appetite. Roughage stimulates peristalsis and bowel movement.

Insufficient roughage in the diet leads to sluggish peristalsis and a tendency to constipation.

Fat Intake

Because of its high food value, fat is an important component of the diet. Furthermore, the palatability of foods is generally enhanced by their content of fat. A molecule of fat is composed of three molecules of fatty acids and one of glycerol. Fats are divided into two groups : animal and vegetable.

Animal Fat : This is found in milk, cheese, butter, eggs, meat, lard, bacon and some fishes like cod, halibut and herring.

Vegetable Fat : This is present in mustard oil, sunflower oil, groundnut oil, cottonseed oil, hydrogenated oils like 'Dalda' and in margarine where vitamins A and D are added. At ordinary levels of intake, 20-25% of the calories of the 1 diet might be derived form fats; for a 3.000 kcal intake, this would represent 66—83 gm of fat. When higher caloric levels are consumed, more fat is likely to be included. An important consideration in lipid nutrition relates to dietary factors influencing blood cholesterol levels. It is now well established that the level of serum cholesterol is decreased by the ingestion of polyunsaturated fatty acids and increased by saturated fatty acids as well as by dietary cholesterol itself.

While there continues to be some disagreement about the relative importance of dietary cholesterol as compared to other factors known to influence the blood cholesterol levels, there is a growing body of evidence supporting the idea that over a certain range of dietary intake the amount of cholesterol ingested does exert a substantial influence on the level of cholesterol in the serum. Mattson and others (1972) have concluded from studies of adult male subjects fed with controlled diets containing 106—317 mg of cholesterol per 1000 kcal that dietary cholesterol can play major role in determining blood cholesterol levels. However, the Indian Heart Association recommends that the energy derived from fats should not exceed 35% of the total daily intake.

Functions of Fat in the Body

(1) *Chief Food Storage Compounds* : Body fat is a reservoir of potential chemical energy. The stored fats in various parts of the body become readily available in times of restricted nutrition for the operation of numerous endergonic process, necessary for the maintenance of life.

(2) *Rich Source of Respiratory Energy* : As a form of energy storage in the body, fat has more than twice the value of protein or carbohydrate, and it is associated with less water in storage. Fatty acids can be used directly as sources of energy by all cells of the body indeed, skeletal muscle and the myocardium appear to utilize fatty acids preferentially as a source of fuel.

(3) *Carriers of Essential Compounds* : The dietary fats serve as the major carriers of the fat-soluble vitamins. A, D, E and K.

(4) *Hormone Synthesis* : Adrenal Corticoids and Sex Hormones are synthesized from fat derivatives.

(5) *Heat Insulation* : Subcutaneous fat in mammals acts as an insulator against excessive heat loss to the environment.

(6) *Structural Components of Cells* : Phospholipids are structural components of cellular membranes, where they contribute to controlling the movement of material into and out of cells.

Protein Requirement

A minimal amount of protein is indispensable in the diet to provide for the replacement of tissue protein, which constantly undergoes destruction and resynthesis. This is often spoken of as the wear-and tear quota. The protein requirement is considerably increased, however, by the demands of growth increased metabolism (as in infection with fever), in burns and after trauma. The requirement for protein in the diet is, however, not only quantitative ; there is also an important qualitative aspect since the metabolism of protein is intimately connected with that of its constituent *amino acids*. These are divided into 2 categories essential and non-essential.

Essential Amino Acids : These amino acids must be obtained preformed -in the diet and cannot be synthesized by the animal organism. A deficiency in any one prevents growth in young animals, and may even cause death. Examples of essential amino acids are *arginine, histidine, isoleucine, leucine, lysine, methionine, phenylalanine thyronine, tryptophan* and *valine.*

Non—Essential Amino Acids : These amino acids are also required by the organism since they are found in the protein of the tissues, but they can apparently be synthesized, presumably from alpha-keto acids, by amination. Examples of non-essential amino adds are *alanine, asparagine, asparatic acid, cystine, glutamic acid, glutamine, glycine, hydroxyproline, proline, serine* and *tyrosine.* Proteins differ in nutritive value depending on their content of essential amino acids. According to this criterion two classes of proteins are recognized: first class and second class proteins.

First Class Proteins : These are the protein foods which contain all of the essential amino acids in the correct proportions. They are obtained almost entirely from animal sources and included : milk eggs meat kidney shellfish milk products poultry fish liver soyabeans

Second Class Proteins : These do not contains all the essential amino acids in the correct proportions, hence called second class proteins. They are derived mainly from vegetable sources. Example are proteins of cereals, root vegetables, nuts and legumes which are known as the pulses. A deficiency of protein among young children is the single most important nutritional problem in the under-developed countries of the world today. The clinical syndrome descriptive of this nutritional deficiency is knows as Kwashiorkar. Besides apamy and loss of appetite, the children suffering from this disease have stunted growth, anaemia, and a protruding abdomen. The victim shows oedema of legs and feet; and changes in the skin and hair colour. Protein malnutrition also result in persistent diarrhoea, loss of weight, and wasting muscles.

Functions of Proteins in the Body

(1) *Structural Components :* Some proteins serve as structural materials of various body parts. Examples of structural proteins are *myosin* of muscles, *keratin* of skin and hair in mammals and *collagen* of connective tissue.

(2) *Biocatalysis (Enzymes) :* The reaction catalyzing enzymes within living cells are all protein of one kind or another.

(3) *Hormones :* Hormones from Pancreatic Islets of Langerhans, Pituitary, Parathyroids and Gastrointestinal mucosa are of *peptide nature.* Similarly, hormones from Thyroid and Adrenal Medulla are derivatives of the amino acid *tyrosine.*

(4) *Blood Constituents :* The dietary proteins provide the amino acids required for the formation of proteins which are present in the blood plasma *i,e., serum albumin serum, globulin, fibrinogen* and *prothrombin. Haemoglobin,* the respiratory pigment in 'rythrocytes, is a conjugated protein composed of colourless basic protein, the *globin* and a pigment *haem. Immunoglobulins* of the blood plasma (β and α —globulins) in mammals and other animals act as *antibodies* that counteract the harmful effects of foreign agents in the body.

(5) *Growth and Repair :* Proteins occupy a key position in the general body growth, and in the repair of wear and tear of the cells with the help of amino acids.

(6) *Food Stuffs :* They provide energy and heat, but only when there is either an insufficiency of carbohydrate in the diet or if it could not be utilized due to deficiency of hormones like insulin. In the latter case, proteins undergo *gluconeogenesis* and are used in cells as food stuffs after getting converted into glucose and glycogen.

Functions and Important Sources of Vitamins

Vitamins	*Best Sources*	*Essential for*	*Deficiancy Symptoms*
Vitamin A *(oil soluble)*	Fish-liver oils, liver and kidney, green and yellow vegetables, yellow fruits, tomatoes, butter, egg yolk.	Growth, health of the eyes, structre and functions of the cells ofthe skin and mucous membranes.	Retarded growth night blindness, susceptibility of skin and membranes, changes in skin and membranes, defective tooth information.
Thiamin (B_1) *(Water soluble)*	Seafood, meat, soyabeans, milk, whole grain, green vegetables fowl.	Growth, carbohydrate and metabolism, functioning of the heart, nerves and muscles.	Retarded growth, loss of appetite and weight, nerve disorders, less resistance to fatige faulty digestion, *(beriberi).*
Riboflavin(B_2 or G) *(Water soluble)*	Meat, soyabeans, milk, green vegetables, eggs, fowl, yeast.	Grwoth, health of skin and mouth, carbohydrate metabolism, functioning of the eyes.	Retarded growth, dimness of vision, inflammation of the tongue premature aging, intolerance to light.
Niacin (B_2) *(water soluble)*	Meat, fowl, fish, peanut, butter, potatoes, whole grain, tomatoes, leafy vegetables.	Growth, carbohydrate metabolism, functioning of the stomach and intestines, functioning of the nervous system.	Smmoothness of the tongue, skin eruptions, digestive distrubances, mental disorders, *(pellagra)*
Vitamin (B_{12}) (water soluble)	Green vagetables, liver.	Preventing pernicious, anemia.	A reduction in number of red blood cells.
Ascorbic acid (C) *(water soluble)*	Coiris fruit, other fruit, tomatoes, leafy vegetables.	Growth, maintaining strength of the bllod vessels, development of teeth, gum health.	Sore gums, hemorrhages around the bones, tendency to bruise easily, *(scurvy).*
Vitamin D *(oil soluble)*	Fish-liver oil, liver,fortified milk, eggs, irradiated foods,	Growth, maintaining strength of the blood vessels, dvelopment of teeth gum health.	Soft bone, poor development of teeth, dental decay, *(reckets).*
Tocopherol (E) *(oil soluble)*	Wheat-germ oil, leafy vegetables, milk, butter.	Normal reproduction.	(Undetermined).
Vitamin K *(oil soluble)*	Green vegetables, soyabean oil, tomatoes.	Normal clotting of the hemorrhages, blood, normal liver functions.	

The Role of Minerals in Human Nutrition

No.	Name	Functions	Important Sources	Effect of Deficiency
1.	Calcium	Most abundant mineral element in the body required for muscle conttraction, normal heart rhythm and nerve irritability. Major constituent of bones and teeth.	Milk, cheese, eggs york, nuts, cabbage, turnip, shrimps.	Poor development of bones dental disorders, stunted growth, rickets in children : may contribute to osteoporosis in adults.
2.	Iron	Constituent of haemoglobin, myoglobin and some oxidative enzymes.	Liver, heart, kidney and spleen are best sources. Other good sources are egg-yolk, nuts, dates, figs, beans, spinach and molasses.	Reduced haemoglobin level and anemia.
3.	Sodium	Participates in the regulation, of muscle and nerve irritability. Regulates osmotic pressure of the extracellular fluids. Buffer salts.	Table salt, meat, fish, milk, eggs and sodium compounds like baking soda and baking powder.	Nausea, muscular cramps, diarrhoea, dehydration.
4.	Patassium	Participates in the regulation of muscle and nerve irritability and affects heart rhythm. Regulates osmotic pressure of intracellular fluid.	Meat, fish, cereals, dried apricotes, banaas, juice of oranges and pineapples and potatoes.	Nervous disoroders, poor muscular control and slow heart rate.
5.	Chlorine	In association with sodium and potassioum, chlorine contributes to maintain normal bodywater content. It is a constituent of gastric juice and maintains acidbase balance.	Table salt, milk, meat, eggs.	Continued vomitting may lead to deficiency followed by alkalisis.

Contd...

No.	Name	Functions	Important Sources	Effect of Deficiency
6.	Phosphours	Major conjstituent of bones teeth. Required for phosphorylation associated with energy-yielding metbolism reactions. Buffer satls.	Milk, cheese, meat, egg-yolk. pulses. nuts and eereals.	Poor mineralization of bones and teeth, rickets, osteomalacis, poor growht.
7.	Iodine	Constituent of thyroid hormones.	In traces as iodides in water, food and common salts. Sea foods and Iodized salt.	Nutritional deficiencny may produce s simplegoitre, low BMR and nervous disorders.
8.	Copper	Required in haemoglobin synthesis, constituent of enzymes like cytochrome oxidase, catalase, uricase, oxidase etc.	Legumes, whole-grain cereals, nuts, liver, meat, fish etc.	Anemia in infants.
9.	Magnesium	Constituent of teeth, bones and many other tissues. Affects muscles and nerve function. Acts on some enzymes of glycolysis.	Cereals, nuts, legumes, cocoa, meat and milk.	Dietary deficiancy not known in man.
10.	Sulphur	Constituent of keratin of hair. Insulin and many proteins.	Eggs, cheese, milk, meat, nuts and pulses.	

Water

Water is not a food but since it is ordinarily consumed in the diet it is included as one of its components. It is a liquid corn-pounds of hydrogen and oxygen in a ratio of 2 : 1. Water plays an Important role in nutrition because it is a constituent of every tissue and cell in the body. Liquid water is an aggregate of hydrogen-bonded clusters of molecules that are continuously forming and breaking up. Hydrogen bond is a non-covalent bond formed by the sharing of a hydrogen bond by two electronegative atoms like oxygens of two water molecules. H-bond is represented by 3 dots.

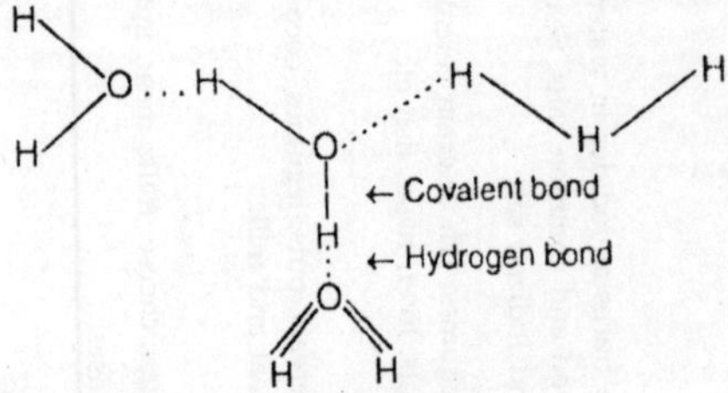

Functions

(1) It acts as a solvent for polar molecules like glucose and for the important salts of sodium, potassium and other minerals necessary in metabolism.

(2) It provides the moist environment which is required by all living cells in the body.

(3) It participates in all the chemical reactions which occur inside and outside the body cells. It is a source of H^+ and OH^- for several biochemical reactions.

(4) As a major component of blood plasma, lymph and the tissue fluid, it transports water soluble substances round the body.

(5) It dilutes and moistens the food.

(6) Water is required for the elimination of excess of salts and waste products which can be dissolved in it.

(7) It helps in the regulation body temperature by the evaporation of sweat from the skin.

(8) It takes part in the formation of urine and faeces.

(9) The biologically active, 3-dimensional conformations of proteins and Nucleic adds are maintained by water.

(10) The arrangement of phospholipids in the lipid bilayers of membranes is carried out by water.

(11) Water helps in maintaining the constancy of internal environment (milieu interior) of the organism. Dibasic phosphate (HPO_4^{2-}), monobasic phosphate ($H_2PO_4^-$) and bicarbonate (HCO_3) remain in solution in the cytoplasm and extracellular fluid. Acids and bases in the body fluids mix with these substances and are neutralized by them.

Recommended Dietary Allowances : In order to simplify the concept of a balanced and adequate diet for normal individuals, foodstuffs have been arranged into our groups, each of which makes a major contribution to the diet. It is recommended that some food from each group be taken daily as specified below :

(1) *Milk Group :* For children, 3 or more 250 ml glasses (smaller servings for some children under 9 years of age) : for teenagers, 4 or more glasses, for adults, or more glasses, cheese, ice cream and other milk products can supply part of the milk recommended.

(2) *Meat Group :* Two or more servings of meat, fish, poultry, eggs or cheese. Dry beans, peas and nuts are alternatives although they cannot substitute entirely or meat, fish, poultry or eggs.

(3) *Vegetable and Fruits :* Four or more servings, including some dark green or yellow vegetable, citrus fruits, or tomatoes. Some uncooked vegetables should be included.

(4) *Breeds and Cereals* : Four or more servings of enriched or whole grain breads and cereals.

Food Intake : The hypothalamus of mammalian brain contains two special eating-control centres which regulate the food intake of the animal. These are called *hunger centre* (H) and *satiety centre* (S) respectively. The two centres function antagonistically to each other when hunger center is stimulated it sends out nerve impulses to various parts of the body that incite the animal to eat. On the other hand, stimulation of satiety centre causes the animal to refuse food. The stimulation of one or the other of these two centres is brought about by the *level of glucose,* in the blood. After eating and digestion subsequently, the glucose concentration in blood tends to rise. High blood glucose level stimulates satiety centre in the brain which inhibits the animal to eat. Conversely long after a meal low blood glucose level stimulates the hunger centre, directing the animal to start food intake.

Adequate glucose delivery to brain depends on various factors such as normal digestion, normal liver function, normal blood circulation, normal hormone balance and normal nervous activities. It is evident, therefore, that *any* disturbance of any body function affects the food intake of the animal.

The Vitamins

Vitamins are complex organic substances found in various foods, which are required for specific metabolic reactions within the cells. In 1912, Dr. Casimir Funk of the Lister Institute of London proposed the name *vitamins* for these *accessory food factors* (Hopkins, 1906). Funk isolated the anti-beriberi substance in pure form from rice polishings. Since the active factor was an amine, and necessary for life, he introduced the term "vitamine". This term has been retained to designate accessory food factors that are neither amino acids nor inorganic elements. Since not all these substances are amines, the term was later modified to *vitamins* by dropping the terminal "e" by Sir J.C. Drummond in 1920, who also proposed their alphabetical nomenclature.

Classification : The vitamins are generally divided into 2 major groups : fat-soluble and water-soluble. The fat-soluble vitamins, which are usually found associated with the lipids of natural foods, include vitamin A, D, E and K. The vitamins of the B complex and vitamin C comprise the water soluble group.

Fat Soluble Vitamins

Vitamin A : It was discovered by McCollum and Davis in 1915.

Chemistry : Vitamin A is a complex primary alcohol, Retinol ($C_{20}H_{29}OH$), which is stored in the animal body in combination with fatty acids, preferrentially the palmitic acid. Retinol represents one half of the β-carotene molecule, the dietary precursor of vitamin A. It is formed by oxidation of the β-carotene molecule at the central; double bond, ending in an alcohol ($—CH_2OH$) group. The vitamin derived in this manner is called vitamin A, which is the most predominant form. Vitamin A (dehydroretinol) is similar to vitamin A, except for an additional double bond in the β-ionone ring.

Metabolic intermediates of vitamin A occur in the form of aldehydes—the retinals, which are important in vision.

Sources : Fish liver oils, butter, whole milk and egg-yolk are foods of animal origin that supply performed vitamin A (retinol). All pigmented (particularly yellow) vegetables and fruits (*e.g.*, sweet potatoes, carrots, pumpkins, papayas, tomatoes, apricots and peaches) and the leafy green vegetables supply provitamin A (carotene) in the diet. Carotenes are precursors to the vitamin in the animal body, β*-carotene* has the highest vitamin A activity and is the most plentiful in human diets. It is an unsaturated hydrocarbon consisting of two six membered rings (β -ionone) and connected by 18 carbon atoms involving nine alternating double bonds. In man, the liver is believed to be the only organ capable of accomplishing the conversion of the cerotenes to vitamin A.

Functions

(1) The maintenance of the integrity of epithelial tissue is an important function of vitamin A. In its absence, normal secretory epithelium is replaced by a dry, koratinized epithelium which is more susceptible to invasion by infectious organisms.

(2) It is essential to growth, particularly of skeleton and other connective tissue.

(3) The retina in most vertebrates contains visual elements consisting of two kinds of light receptors —*rods* and *cones*. The rods are concerned with vision in dim light (night vision) and the cones are the organs of vision in bright light (day vision) and of colour vision. Vitamin A is a constituent of "visual purple" *rhodopsin,* a photo-sensitive pigment of the rod cells and of *iodopsin* in the cones of retina. The specific role of vitamin A in the physiologic mechanism of vision has been elucidated largely by Wald and Morton.

(4) It prevents infection.

(5) Vitamin A helps in keeping normal fertility.

Deficiencies of Vitamin A (Avitaminosis)

(1) *Night blindness (nyctalopia),* which is a disturbance of rod vision, is one manifestation of vitamin A deficiency.

(2) *Xerophthalmia, i. e.,* Keratinization of ocular tissue, which may progress to blindness, is a late result of vitamin A deficiency. Xerophthalmia is a major cause of blindness in childhood. It is still a major health problem

in many parts of the world, especially in Hong Kong, Manila, Saigon and Dacca.

(3) In the absence of vitamin A, the growth of experimental animals does not progress normally. The skeleton is affected first, and then the soft tissues.

(4) In the growing animal; collagenous tissues are particularly affected by a deficiency of vitamin A.

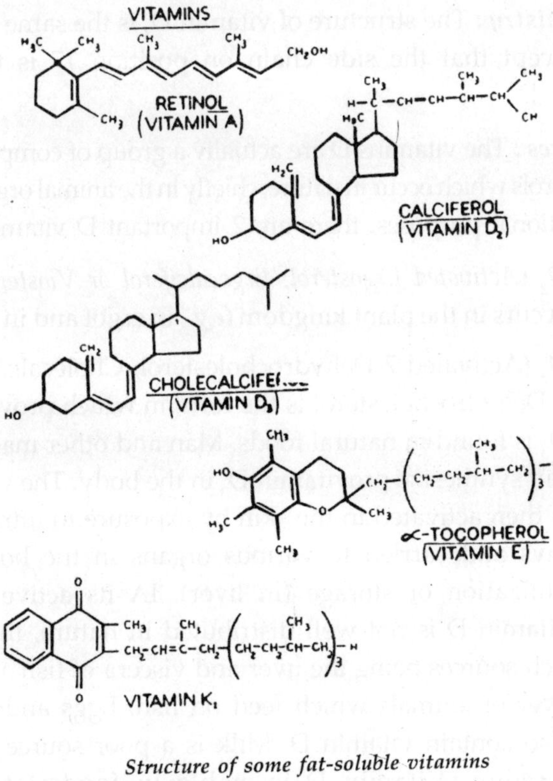

Structure of some fat-soluble vitamins

Toxicity of Vitamin A : *Hypervitaminosis A* may occur as a consequence of the administration of large doses (in the form of vitamin A concentrates) of infants and small children. The principal symptoms are painful joints, periosteal thickening of long bones, and loss of hair. Preformed vitamin A in large amounts may be toxic to adults as well as children.

Vitamin D : In 1921, Mellanby recognized the need for a factor in food (cod liver oil) that could prevent rickets. McCollum demonstrated that this vitamin was not the same as vitamin A, and in 1924, Steenbock and Hess were able to show that many foods acquire vitamin D activity after exposure to ultraviolet irradiation.

Chemistry : The structure of vitamin D_3 is the same as that of D_2 except that the side chain on position 17 is that of cholesterol.

Sources : The vitamins D are actually a group of compounds. All are sterols which occur in nature, chiefly in the animal organism. For nutritional purposes, there are 2 important D vitamins :

(i) *D_2 (Activated Ergosterol; Ergocalciferol or Viosterol) :* It occurs in the plant kingdom (*e.g.*, in ergot and in yeast).

(ii) D_3 (Activated 7-Dehydrocholesterol, Cholecalciferol) : 7-Dehydrocholesterol is the form in which provitamin D_3 is found in natural foods. Man and other mammals can synthesize provitamin D_3 in the body. The vitamin is then activated in the skin by exposure to ultraviolet rays and carried to various organs in the body for utilization or storage (in liver). IA its active form, vitamin D is not well distributed in nature, the only rich sources being the liver and viscera of fish and the liver of animals which feed on fish. Eggs and butter also contain vitamin D. Milk is a poor source of the vitamin. Vitamin D is stable in foods; storage, processing, and cooking do not effect its activity.

Functions : The principal action of Vitamin D is to regulate the absorption and utilization of calcium and phosphorus. The vitamin also has a direct effect on the calcification process.

Deficiency

(1) *Rickets in children* : Slow growth, degenerate calcium metabolism and deformed bones (*e.g.*, bowlegs, knock-knees, enlarged joints, rachitic rosary — a beaded appearance of the ribs and "pigeon breast").

(2) *Osteomalacia* (soft bones) in some adults, particularly in women during pregnancy.

Toxicity of Vitamin D : Excessive quantities of vitamin D (ten times the normally required daily level) given over prolonged periods either to children or to adults produce demineralization of bone, and multiple fractures may occur after only minimal trauma. Serum calcium and phosphorus are both markedly elevated, resulting in metastatic calcification of many soft tissues and formation of renal calculi. The latter may block the renal tubules sufficiently to cause a secondary hydronephrosis.

Vitamin E : In 1936, Evans and Emerson isolated vitamin E from wheat-germ oil. It was given the name *tocopherol* (Gk. *tokos,* childbirth ; *phero,* to bear ; *ol,* an alcohol).

Chemistry : The tocopherols are unsaturated alcohols. There are 4 varieties of tocopherols : alpha, beta, gamma and delta tocopherol ; of these, alpha tocopherol ($C_{29}H_{50}O_2$) has the widest distribution and greatest biological activity. It has a "chromane ring system" containing four methyl (—CH_3) groups, one phenolic group and a phytyl side chain. The beta and gamma tocopherols have one methyl group less in the ring than α-tocopherol.

Sources : The richest natural sources of tocopherol are plant oils, *e.g.* wheatgerm, rice, cotton seed, as well as the lipids of green leaves. Fish-liver oils, rich in vitamins A and D, are devoid of tocopherol. Good sources of vitamin E include eggs, muscle meats, liver, fish and chicken.

Functions

(1) The most striking chemical characteristic of the vitamin E is their antioxidant property. Polyunsaturated fatty acids are easily attacked by molecular oxygen, resulting in the formation of peroxides. The tocopherols prevent this.

(2) It is required for the normal reproductive function in rats, hence also called "antisterility" vitamin. In the absence of vitamin E, the germinal epithelium of the testes of rats is destroyed. In the female rat, ovulation and fertilization take place, but there is death and resorption of the foetus. This situation can be repaired by including vitamin E in the diet.

(3) In some animal *e.g.*, rabbit a lack of vitamin E produces muscular dystrophy.

Deficiency : The wide distribution of vitamin E in vegetable oils, cereal grains, and animal fats makes it unlikely that a deficiency of this nutrient occurs in normal humans.

Vitamin K : *(Koagulations* vitamin) was identified is 1935 by Dam as a factor present in green leaves which prevented haemorrhage.

Chemistry : The vitamin isolated from alfalfa is called vitamin K_1 (Phylloquinone). It is a derivative of 2-methyl –1, 4-naphthoquinone with a phytyl radical on position 3. Another compound with antihaemophilic properties was isolated from bacteria and called vitamin K_2 (Farnoquinone).

Sources : Vitamin K is present in alfalfa and in such dark green vegetables as spinach, cabbage leaves as well as in cauliflower and peas. Tomatoes, cheese, egg-yolk, and liver are good sources. Fruits are poor sources, as are moulds, yeast and fungi.

Functions : The best known function of vitamin K is to catalyze the synthesis of prothrombin by the liver. It also regulates the synthesis of other plasma clotting factors dependent on vitamin K (factor VII, IX and X).

Deficiency : In the absence of vitamin K a hypoprothrombinemia occurs in which blood clotting time may be greatly prolonged. A dietary deficiency of vitamin K is not likely to occur since the vitamin is fairly well distributed in foods and the intestinal micro-organisms synthesize considerable vitamin K in the intestine. However, a deficiency may occur as a result of prolonged oral therapy with drugs capable of vitamin K-producing bacteria (Sulfaguanidine). Furthermore, the absorption of vitamin K from the intestine depends on the presence of bile. A deficiency state will therefore result as a consequence of biliary tracts obstruction or if there is a defect in fat absorption, such as in sprue and celiac disease.

Water Soluble Vitamins

Vitamins of the 'B' Complex Thiamine (B_1) (Antiberiberi substance, Antineuritic factor) : The structure of thiamine, which was first isolated in crystalline form by Jansen and Windaus in 1926, was established by Williams and his coworkers in 1936.

Chemistry : Thiamin ($C_{12}H_{17}N_4OS$) is 2, 5-diemthyl-6-aminopyrimidine bonded through a methylene linkage to 4-methyl–5–hydroxyl–ethyl–thiazole.

Sources : The outer layers of the seeds of plants are especially rich in thiamine. Whole-wheat bread, therefore, is an excellent source, whereas ordinary white bread is a poor source of the vitamin, since most of the thiamine is removed in the milling process. Among the more abundant sources are unrefined cereal grains, legumes, brewer's yeast, liver, kidney and lean cuts of pork. Excessive cooking leaches the water-soluble thiamine from many food stuffs.

Functions : It is a constituent of the coenzyme *thiamine pyrophosphate* (TPP) and is essential for carbohydrate metabolism (oxidative decarboxylation of pyruvate or of α–ketoglutarate).

Deficiency : Thiamine deficiency causes *Beriberi* which was first described by Admiral Takaki in 1887 among Japanese sailors. The disease is still an important public health problem in Philippines, Vietnam, Thailand and Burma where polished milled rice is a staple food. Beriberi affects predominantly the peripheral nervous system, the gastrointestinal tract and the cardiovascular system. There are two forms of the disease: "dry" and "wet" beriberi. In the dry form, there is rapid loss of weight and muscle wasting. Marked peripheral neuritis and muscular weakness result in the patient's becoming almost helpless. Deep reflexes are lost, sensory changes may occur, and anxiety states and mental confusion are evident. The heart becomes enlarged. In wet beriberi, there is a generalized oedema that may obscure the weakness and muscular wasting. Acute cardiac symptoms may develop rapidly.

Riboflavin (B_2) : Warburg and Christian isolated this *yellow enzyme* from yeast in 1932.

Chemistry : Riboflavin corresponds to 6, 7-dimethyl-9-ribiryl-isoalloxa-zine and contains the alcohol (ribitol) derived from the sugar ribose attached at position 9.

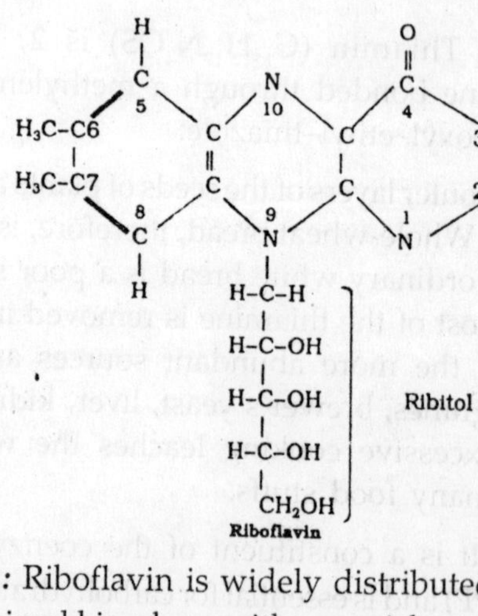

Riboflavin

Sources : Riboflavin is widely distributed throughout the plant and animal kingdom, with very rich sources in anaerobic fermenting bacteria. Milk, liver, kidney, and heart are excellent sources. Many vegetables are also good sources, but the cereals are rather low in riboflavin content.

Functions : It is a constituent of two coenzymes—flavin mono-nucleotide (FMN), and flavin adenine dinucleotide (FAD), which are involved in intermediary metabolism. All known biological functions of riboflavin involve these two coenzymes.

Deficiency : Riboflavin deficiency in man is characterized by a particular type of glossitis (magenta-coloured tongue), fissures at the corners of the mouth and lips (cheilosis), localized seborrheic dermatitis of the face and corneal vascularization.

Nicotinic Acid or Niacin

Pellagra-preventing, PP, factor of Goldberger : Pellagra was recognized as early as 1735 by Caspar Casal, physician to Philip V of Spain. The identification of nicotinic acid as the responsible factor was made by Elvehjem, Woolley, and their associates in 1937.

Chemistry : Nicotinic acid or Niacin is pyridine–3–carboxylic acid. Its amide is nicotinamide.

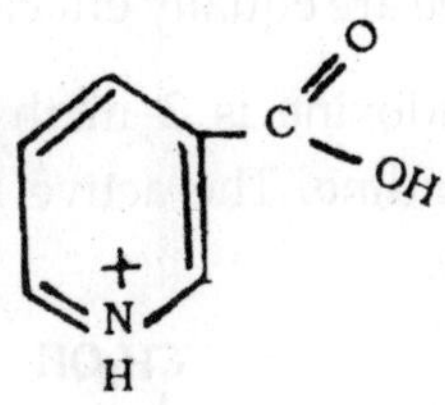

Nicotinic Acid

Sources : Niacin is found most abundantly in yeast. Lean meats, liver, and poultry are good sources. Milk, tomatoes, canned salmon, and several leafy green vegetables contribute sufficient amounts of the vitamin to prevent disease. Body can synthesize this vitamin from the amino acid tryptophan.

Functions : It is convertible into nicotinamide and thus functions metabolically as a component of the 2 coenzymes: nicotinamide adenine dinucleotide (NAD) and nicotinamide adenine dinucleotide phosphate (NADP). These coenzymes, which operate as hydrogen and electron transfer agents by virtue of reversible oxidation and reduction, play a vital role in metabolism, leading to the formation of ATP in the electron transport system (ETS).

Deficiency : *Pellagra* was established as a deficiency disease by Goldberger. The disease is symptomatized by three D's, namely diarrhoea, dermatitis of those areas that are exposed to sunlight and dementia, due to disturbances of the central nervous system. Stomatitis and glossitis are also associated with the other symptoms. Alcoholism causes deficiency of the vitamin and is an important precipitating factor of the disease.

Pyridoxal/Pyridoxamine/Pyridoxine

(B_6 Group) (Rat Antidermatitis Factor) : Pyridoxine was first discovered in 1938 and synthesized by Stiller in 1939. Natural sources contain two other forms of this vitamin, pyridoxal and pyridoxamine. The three substances as a group are designated vitamin B_6 ; no single one is considered the vitamin, since all three are equally effective in animal nutrition.

Chemistry : Pyridoxine is 2–methyl–3–hydroxy –4, 5–di (hydroxymethyl) pyridine. The active form of the vitamin is pyridoxal phosphate.

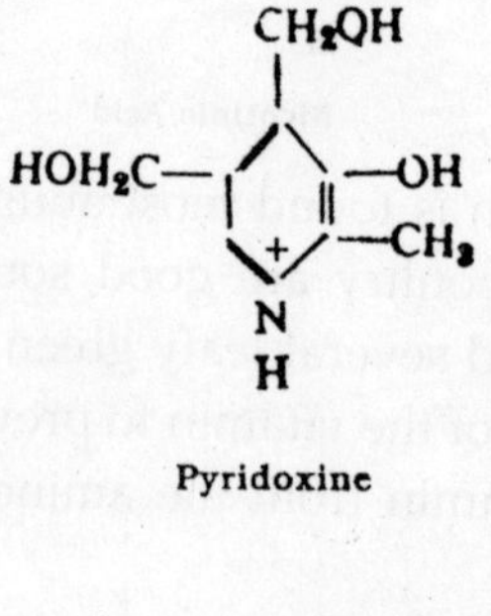

Pyridoxine

Sources : The B_6 group is widely distributed in nature, and those foods rich in other members of the B complex are excellent sources of these materials, *e.g.*, the germs of various grains and seeds, egg yolk, yeast and meat, particularly liver and kidney.

Functions

(1) It is a constituent of coenzymes *pyridoxal phosphate*, which is involved in the non-oxidative degradation of amino acids, viz., transamination, deamination, decarboxylation etc.

(2) It is essential in the synthesis of haem for haemoglobin and cytochromes.

Deficiency : There is little evidence that diets containing a reasonable balance of naturally occurring foodstuffs are ever seriously deficient in vitamin B_6. However, occasional cases of B_6 deficiency do arise as a result of malabsorption, alcoholism, antagonism to drugs etc. Pyridoxine deficiency in humans may be associated with a reversible hypochromic microcytic anemia with a high serum iron similar to that observed in pyridoxine deficient animals.

Pantothenic Acid (B_5) : This factor was first recognized as a portion of the "bios" complex by R.J. Williams and his colleagues in 1933. The significance of this substance in animal nutrition was established by Jukes, Woolley, and their associates.

Chemistry : Pantothenic acid is N–(α, γ–dihydroxy–β, β-dimethyl– butyryl) β-aminopropionic acid. It was isolated from yeast.

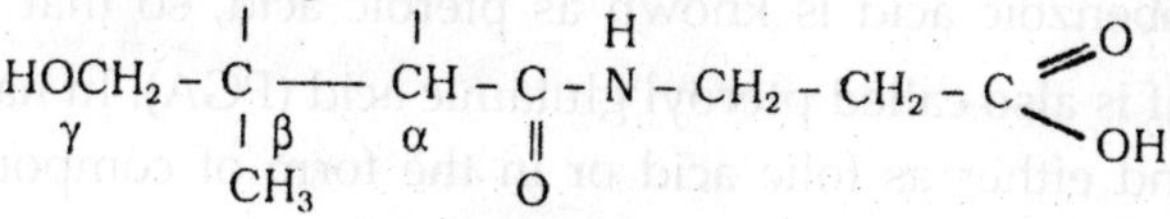

Pantothenic Acid

Sources : Pantothenic acid is widely distributed in food, particularly in that from animal sources, in whole grain cereals, and in legumes. Excellent food sources include egg yolk, kidney, liver, and yeast. Lean beef, skimmed milk, sweet potatoes, and molasses are fair sources. Royal jelly, prepared by the bee colony for the nutrition of the queen bee, and fish ovaries before spawning are the richest known sources of this vitamin.

Functions : In its active form, pantothenic acid is a constituent of *coenzyme A,* which is essential to several fundamental reactions in metabolism. An example is the combination of coenzyme A with acetate to form acetyl-coenzyme A which participates in a number of important metabolic processes like citric acid cycle. Besides, acetyl-CoA is a precursor of cholesterol and thus of the steroid hormones.

Deficiency : Pantothenic acid deficiency causes gastrointestinal disturbances, skin symptoms such as cornification, depigmentation, desquamation etc. Lack of this vitamin also affects the adrenals.

Folic Acid Folacin or Pteroylglutamic Acid (Pga) Vitamin M/Vitamin B_1 Bitamin B_{10} : Existence of this nutritional factor was first suggested by Day. It was named folic acid by Mitchell, Snell and Williams, because potent concentrates were obtained from spinach leaf *(L. foliwri).* The chemical structure was established in 1945.

Chemistry : It is a combination of glutamic acid, β-aminobenzoic acid, and a pteridine. Pteridine bound to β-aminobenzoic acid is known as pteroic acid, so that folic acid itself is also called pteroyl glutamic acid (PGA). In nature it is found either as folic acid or in the form of compounds containing additional glutamic acid residues.

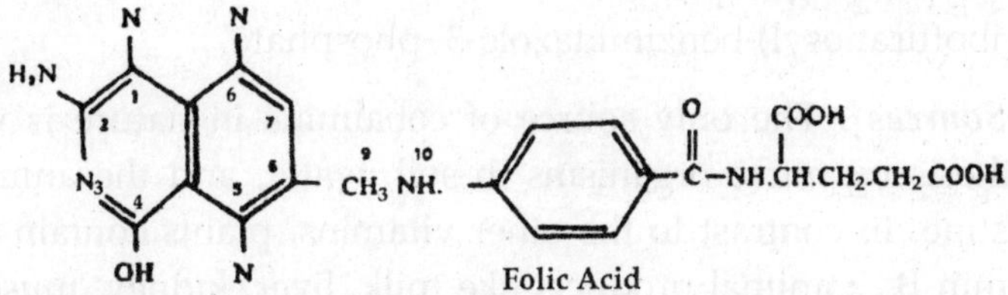

Folic Acid

Sources : The richest sources of the vitamin are yeast, liver, kidney, and green vegetables, with moderate amounts contained in dairy foods, meat and fish. There is very little in fruits.

Functions

(1) The folic acid coenzymes are specifically concerned with biochemical reactions involving the transfer and utilization of the single carbon (C–l) moiety.

(2) The folic acid participates in reactions leading to synthesis of purines and thymine required for DNA synthesis.

(3) It takes part in the formation and maturation of red blood cells.

Deficiency : Folic acid deficiency is characterized by growth failure, sprue, macrocytic anemia of pregnancy, certain marcocytic anemias of children and leukopenia.

Cyanacobalamin (B_{12})

Cobamide Cyanide, Antipernicious Anaemia Factor, Cobalmin : Vitamin B_{12}, the anti-pernicious anemia factor (extrinsic factor of Castle) was first isolated by Smith and Parker in 1948 from liver as a red crystalline compound containing cobalt and phosphorus.

Chemistry : Vitamin B_{12} is a darkred compound containing one atom of cobalt that is bound by coordinate linkages to the four nitrogen atoms of a partially hydrogenated tetrapyrrole, to a cyanide group and to a nucleotide : 5, 6-dimethyl-l-(D-ribofuranosyl)-benzimidazole-3'-phosphate.

Sources : The only source of cobalmins in nature is via synthesis by micro-organisms in soil, water, and the animal intestine. In contrast to the other vitamins, plants contain no vitamin B_{12} ; animal products like milk, liver, kidney, muscle meat, eggs and cheese are the primary dietary sources of the vitamin.

Functions

(1) It is necessary for the maturation of erythrocytes in the red bone marrow.

(2) As a component of the various coenzymes, vitamin B_{12} has its greatest effect on nucleic acid formation.

(3) It is important for the maintenance of normal health and activity of certain parts of the nervous system.

(4) The vitamin B_{12} coenzyme has been shown to catalyze the isomerase reaction in animal tissue. By this reaction, methylmalonyl-CoA is converted to succinyl-CoA.

(5) It has a role in transmethylation process.

Absorption of Vitamin B_{12} : Vitamin B_{12} is absorbed from the ileum, but its absorption is dependent upon the presence of HCl and a constituent of normal gastric juice designated *intrinsic factor* (IF) by castle. Human intrinsic factor is a mucoprotein that binds one molecule of vitamin B_{12} per molecule of protein. The gastric parietal cells are the source of both HCl acid and intrinsic factor in man.

Deficiency : The most characteristic sign of a deficiency of vitamin B_{12} in man is the development of *pernicious* or *macrocytic anemia*. In this form of anemia, the blood cells are larger than normal (hence the term 'macrocytic'), but fewer in number. Instead of 5 million red cells/cu mm., the count may drop to

1 million cu. mm. only. Pernicious anemia results not from inadequate ingestion of vitamin B_{12}, but from an inadequate secretion of "intrinsic factor" in the gastric juice, which promotes the absorption of ingested vitamin B_{12} from the intestine. The latter is an essential factor for the formation and maturation of RBC's. Symptoms of pernicious anemia include numbness and tingling of the hands and feet, nervousness, a sore and smooth tongue and poor appetite.

Biotin

In 1936, Kogl and Tonnis isolated from egg-yolk a crystalline growth factor for yeast, which they named 'biotin'.

Chemistry : ' Biotin ($C_{10}H_{16}O_3N_2S$) is hexahydro-2-oxo-l-thieno-3, 4-imidazole-4-valeric acid.

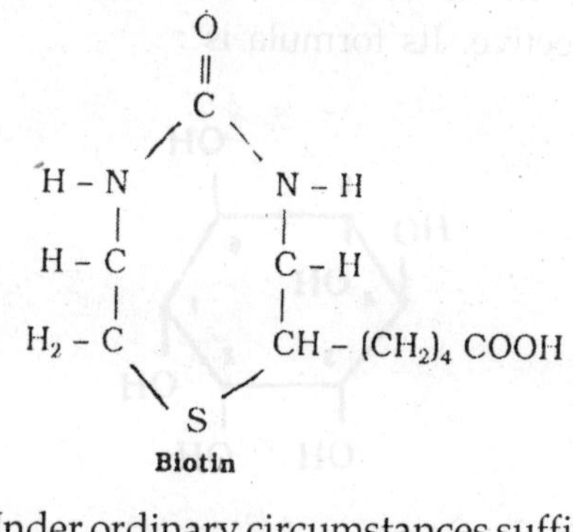

Biotin

Sources : Under ordinary circumstances sufficient quantities of biotin are provided to the mammal by intestinal becterial synthesis. The vitamin is widely distributed in natural foods. Egg-yolk, kidney, liver, tomatoes, and yeast are excellent sources. Pea-nuts and chocolate contain abundant quantities.

Functions : In biological system, biotin functions as the coenzyme for *carboxyloses,* enzymes which catalyze carbon dioxide "fixation" or carboxylation.

Deficiency : Biotin deficiency cannot be produced in most animals merely by diets deficient in this nutrient, presumably because of intestinal bacterial synthesis of this compound. However, biotin deficiency has been produced in poultry, monkeys and rats on synthetic rations. Biotin deficiency follows either sterilization of the intestinal tract, the feeding of raw egg-white, or the administration of biotin antimetabolites.

In experiments with rats, dermatitis, retarded growth, loss of hair, and loss of muscular control occurred when egg-white was fed as the sole source of protein. Raw egg-white contains a glycoprotein *avidin* which antagonises biotin and thus the animals suffers from deficiency of this vitamin.

Inositol

There are 9 isomers of inositol. *Myo-inositol* is the most important one in nature and the only isomer which is biologically effective. Its formula is :

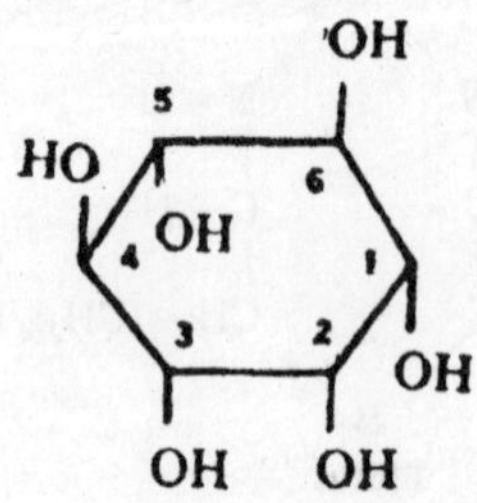

Myo-Inositol

Sources : Inosito l is found in fruits, meat, milk, nuts, vegetables, wholegrains and yeast.

Functions : The significance of this compound in human nutrition has not been established. Together with choline inositol, has a lipotropic action in experimental animals.

Deficiency : Deficiency symptoms in mice include so-called spectacled eye, alopecia, and failure of lactation and growth.

Choline

Choline is an important metabolite, although probably it cannot be classified as a vitamin since it is synthesized by the body.

$$HO—CH_2—CH_2—N^+—(CH_3)_3$$

Acetylcholine, produced from choline and acetic acid, is well known as a chemical mediator of parasympathetic as well as certain other types of activity in the nervous systems. *Acetylcholine-esterase* is an enzyme, present in many tissues which hydrolyzes acetylcholine to choline and acetic acid.

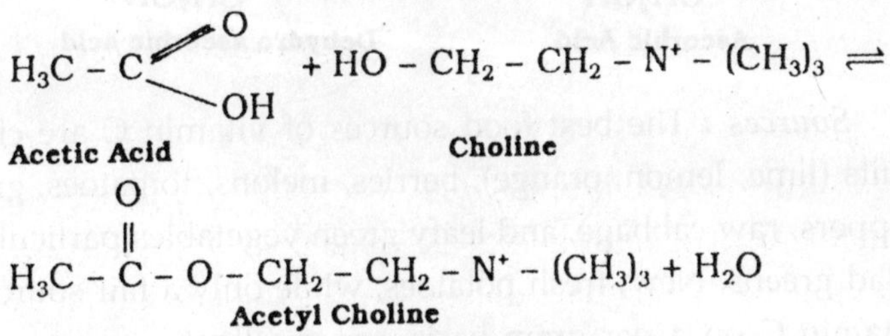

Acetyl Choline

In many animal species, a deficiency of choline leads to the development of fatty livers causing disturbances in fat metabolism. In the young growing rat there is also hemorrhagic degeneration of the kidneys.

Vitamin C (Ascorbic acid, Antiscorbutic Vitamin) : In 1753, Captain James Lind of the British Navy showed that the disease *Scurvy* which was common is sailors could be cured by giving them Lemons and oranges. In 1907 Hoist and Frolich demonstrated that guinea pigs develop scorbutic lesions on a diet of oats and bran. The vitamin was isolated by Szent-Gyorgyi (1928) from orange juice. In 1932, King and Waugh isolated the crystalline vitamin, which had previously been termed vitamin C and has been renamed ascorbic acid.

Chemistry : The chemical structure of vitamin C resembles that of a monosaccharide. Vitamin C is chemically known as ascorbic acid. It can be readily oxidised to the dehydro form.

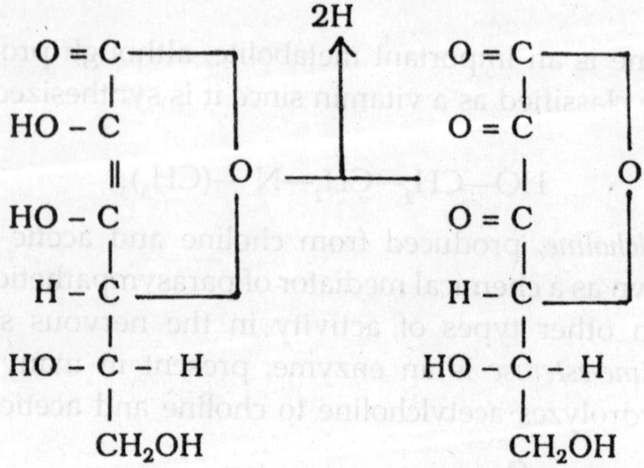

Ascorbic Acid **Dehydro ascorbic acid**

Sources : The best food sources of vitamin C are citrus fruits (lime, lemon, orange), berries, melons, tomatoes, green peppers, raw cabbage, and leafy green vegetables particularly salad greens. New, fresh potatoes, while only a fair source of Vitamin C on a per gram basis, are excellent sources in the average diet because of the quantities which are commonly used. Animal sources are generally poor except the adrenal cortex.

The vitamin is easily destroyed by cooking, since it is readily oxidised. Mincing of fresh vegetables such as cabbage, mashing of potatoes, canning and other food- preparation procedures may destroy a portion of the ascorbic acid in foods.

Functions : Both forms are physiologically active, and both are found in the body fluids.

(1) Maintains the normal intracellular material of cartilage; dentine and bone ; and the integrity of capillary walls.

(2) Has a specific role in collagen synthesis.

(3) Provides resistance against common colds and infections.

(4) Helps to dissolve cholesterol in blood.

(5) Plays an important role in wound repair and activates metabolism.

(6) Protects the body against stress.

(7) Enhances the absorption of iron from vegetables, cereals and fruits.

Deficiency : It has long been known that smoking lowers the body's store of vitamin C, and that pregnant and breast-feeding women need more of it. It is also known that those eating institutional food, which is kept hot for long periods, tend to fall short of vitamins.

Severe vitamin C deficiency produces *Scurvy.* The pathological signs of this disease are skin eruptions, swollen bleeding gums, loosening of the teeth, haemorrhages, poor healing of wounds, easy fractures of bones and increased susceptibility to infections.

The infant is usually well supplied with vitamin C at birth. However, infants 6–12 months of age who are fed processed milk formulas, not supplemented with fruits and vegetables, are very susceptible to the development of *infantile scurvy.* Elderly bachelors and widowers who may prepare their own foods are particularly prone to the development of vitamin C deficiency, a syndrome termed "bachelor scurvy."

Dr. R. Elwyn Hughes, writing in the Nutrition Foundation booklet, "Vitamin C—some Current Problems", recommends 70–100 mg daily in most cases with a marginal increase to 100-130 mg for special cases like slimmers, the elderly, and heavy smokers. Noble Prize winner biochemist Dr. Linus Pauling has always argued that huge doses *(i. e.,* hundreds of mg daily, not between 30 or 100) can perform curative miracles.

Recommended Daily Requirements of Vitamins in Humans

		Fat-Soluble Vitamins				Water-Soluble Vitamins							
	Age (years)	Weight (kg)	Vitamin A Actiuitiy (U)	Vitamin D (IU)	Vitamin E Activity (IU)	Ascorbic Acid (mg)	Folacin (mcg)	Niacin (mg)	Ribo-flavin (mg)	Thia-min (mg)	Vitamin B_6 (mg)	(B_{12}) (mcg)
Infants	0.0–0.5	5	2000	500	5	35	50	10	0.4	0.3	0.3	0.3
	0.5–1.0	8	2500	500	6	35	50	16	0.6	0.5	0.4	0.3
Children	1–3	12	2500	500	8	40	100	18	0.8	0.7	0.6	1.0
	4–6	18	3000	500	10	40	200	24	2.0	1.5	0.9	1.5
	7–10	25	3800	500	13	45	300	32	2.5	2.5	1.2	2.0
Males	11–14	40	6000	400	16	50	500	36	3.00	2.5	1.6	3.0
	15–18	50	6000	400	16	50	500	40	3.00	2.5	2.0	3.0
	19–22	55	6000	400	16	50	500	40	3.00	2.5	2.0	3.0
	23–50	65	6000		16	50	500	36	2.5	2.–3	2.0	3.0
	51	65	6000		13	50	500	32	2.5	2.2	2.0	3.0
Females	11–14	40	5000	400	13	50	500	32	2.0	1.8	1.6	3.0
	15–18	45	5000	400	13	50	500	28	2.0	1.8	2.0	3.0
	19–22	48	5000	400	13	50	500	28	2.0	1.8	2.0	3.0
	23–50	55	5000		13	50	500	26	2.0	1.8	2.0	3.0
	51*	55	5000		13	50	500	24	2.0	1.8	2.0	3.0
Pregnant			6000	700	16	75	8000	+2	+0.5	+.5	2.5	4.0
Lactating			7000	700	16	100	800	+4	+1.0	+.8	2.5	4.0

* One International (Unit) (IU) of Vitamin D corresponds to 0.000025 milligram.

The Proteins

The name *protein* derived from the Greek word *proteios,* which means "of the first rank" was coined by Berzelius in 1838 to emphasize the importance of this class of complex nitrogenous substances found in the cells of animals and plants. Proteins occupy a central position in the architecture and functioning of living matter.

The chemical and physical activity that constitutes the life of the cell, is catalyzed by *enzymes,* all of which are proteins. Some proteins serve as structural, extracellular elements, for examples as *hair, wool* and the *collagen* of connective tissue. Other proteins may be *hormones* or *oxygen-carriers,* participate in muscular contraction, are associated with the genes and are concerned with immunological defense mechanisms as *antibodies* etc. Proteins are qualitatively the main material of animal tissue, for they may constitute as much as 3/4 of the dry substance.

Proteins are Built from Amino Acids : Chemically, proteins are polymers of molecular units called *amino acids.* For this reason, the amino acids are referred to as the "building blocks" of proteins. These polymers contain, carbon, hydrogen, oxygen and nitrogen atoms. Sulphur atoms are usually present too. Certain proteins contain phosphorus or some trace metal elements, such as copper or iron, in addition to the other elements. The proteins have high molecular weights ranging from 5,000 to many millions. Each is a *macromolecule :* The repeating units are the amino acids, of which 20 are commonly found in proteins, and are linked together by peptide bonds. A protein molecule consists of one or more polypeptide chains, each chain containing from approximately 20 to several hundred amino acid residues.

General Chemical Composition of the Amino Acids : The same 20 amino acids have been found in the proteins of all species of microorganisms, plants and animals. Several additional amino acids are limited distribution and occur in only one or a few kinds of proteins. The general structure of an amino acid is represented by the formula.

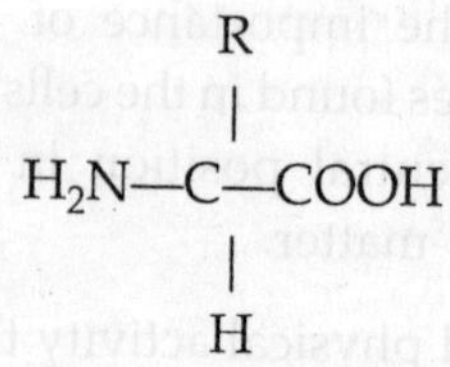

Where $-NH_2$ is an amino group, -COOH a carboxylic group, and -R an organic group, referred to as a *side chain,* which varies in structure from one amino acid to the other. The side chain may be *polar* or *non-polar.*

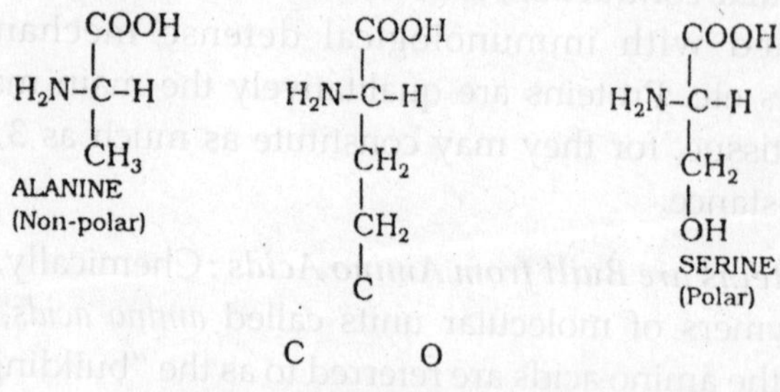

Glutamic Acid (Glutamate) Polar

The carbon atom to which R group is bonded is called the α -carbon. The simplest amino acid is *glycine,* where R = H. If R = CH_3, the amino acid is *alanine,* and if R = CH_2OH, the acid is called *serine.* Many other amino acids are characterized by comparatively more complex —R groups. They are either in the form of carbon chains, both straight and branched, or are rings.

The amino acids present in proteins have both an amino and a carboxylic group attached to the same (a) carbon atom; hence they are described as α -amino acids.

A free amino group at the end of the side chain is basic, a free carboxyl group is acidic.

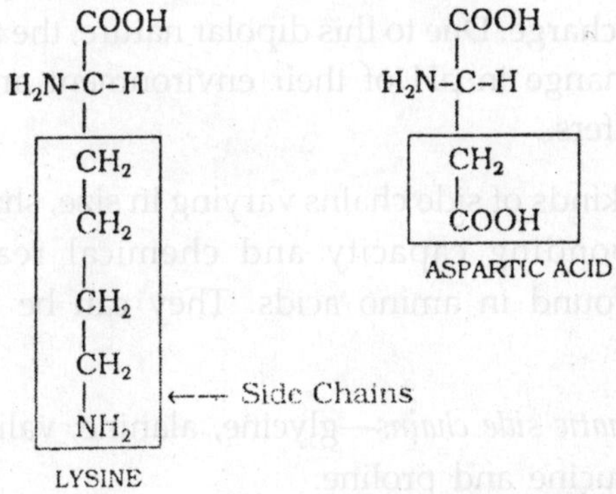

Lysine and *Arginine* have two amino (NH_2) groups and one carboxyl (COOH) group, hence they are Basic amino acids. *Glutamic acid* (Glutamate) and *Aspartic acid* (aspartate) contain one NH_2 and two COOH groups each, hence called Acidic amino acids. *Glycine, Alanine, Valine* and *Phenylcdanine* are neutral amino acids because they contain one NH_2 and one COOH group.

Amphoteric Properties

Since amino acids contains both amino (–NH_2 and corboxylic (–COOH) groups, they may act as weak alkali bases or as weak acids. COOH group may dissociate and yield H^+ whereas -NH_2 group of the same compound may accept the H^+.

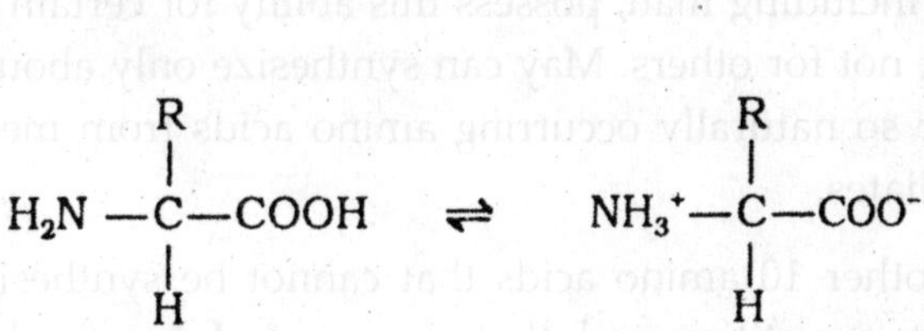

Substances possessing this dual property are called *amphoteric compounds, dipolar ions or zwitter ions* (GK, *zwitter*, hermaphrodite). In the dipolar form of an amino acid, the amino group is protonated (—NH_3^+) and the carboxyl group is dissociated (—COO^-). Although charged, the zwitter ion bears no net charge. Due to this dipolar nature, the amino acids resist any change in pH of their environment and can thus serve as buffers.

Twenty kinds of side chains varying in size, shape, charge, hydrogen bonding capacity and chemical reactivity are commonly found in amino acids. They can be grouped as follows :

(a) *Aliphatic side chains*—glycine, alanine, valine, leucine, isoleucine and proline.

(b) *Hydroxyl aliphatic side chains*—serin and threonine.

(c) *Aromatic side chains*—phenylalanine, tyrosine and tryptophan.

(d) *Basic side chains*—lysine, arginine and histidine.

(e) *Acidic side chains*—aspartic acid and glutamic acid.

(f) *Amide side chains*—asparagine and glutamine.

(g) *Sulfur side chains*—cysteine and methionine.

Essential and Nonessential Amino Acids : Most prokaryotic cells, *(e.g.,* bacteria) and many eukaryotic cells, *(e.g.,* plants, yeasts) are capable of synthesizing from amphibolic intermediates, all the amino acids present in proteins. Higher animals, including man, possess this ability for certain amino acids but not for others. May can synthesize only about 10 of the 20 or so naturally occurring amino acids from metabolic intermediates.

The other 10 amino acids that cannot be synthesized in sufficient quantities and that are needed for the normal functioning of the animal are called *nutritionally essential amino acids*. These must be obtained from the diet ; a deficiency in any one prevents growth in young animals, and may even cause death. Animals must, therefore, consume daily doses of essential amino acids. Those amino acids that can be synthesized from amphibolic intermediates are designed *nutritionally non-essential amino acids.*

Essential and Non-essential Amino Acids

Essential; must be supplied preformed in dietary proteins	*Non-essential; may be synthesized by the tissue*
Arginine* (Arg)	Alanine (Ala)
Histidine* (His)	Asparagine (Asn)
Isoleucine (Ile)	Aspartic acid (Asp)
Leucine (Leu)	Cyteine (Cys)
Lysine (Lys)	Glutamic acid (Glu)
Methionine (Met)	Glutamine (Gix)
Phenylalanine (Phe)	Glycine (Gly)
Threonine (Thr)	Proline (Pro)
Tryptophan (Trp)	Serine (Ser)
Valine (Val)	Tyrosine (Tyr)

*Arginine and histidine are sometimes classified as "semi-essential" because, they may be synthesized in the tissues but not at adequate rates to support growth in younger human individuals.

Proteins are Built from a Stock of Twenty Amino Acids

Amino acid	*Three letter Abbreviation*
Alanine	Ala
Arginine	Arg
Asparagine	Asn
Aspartic acid	Asp
Cysteine	Cys
Glutamine	Gln
Glutamic acid	Glu
Glycine	Gly
Histidine	His
Isoleucine	Ile
Leucine	Leu
Lysine	Lys
Methionine	Met

Contd...

Amino acid	*Three letter Abbreviation*
Phenylalanine	Phe
Proline	Pro
Serine	Ser
Threonine	Thr
Tryptophan	Trp
Tyrosine	Tyr
Valine	Val

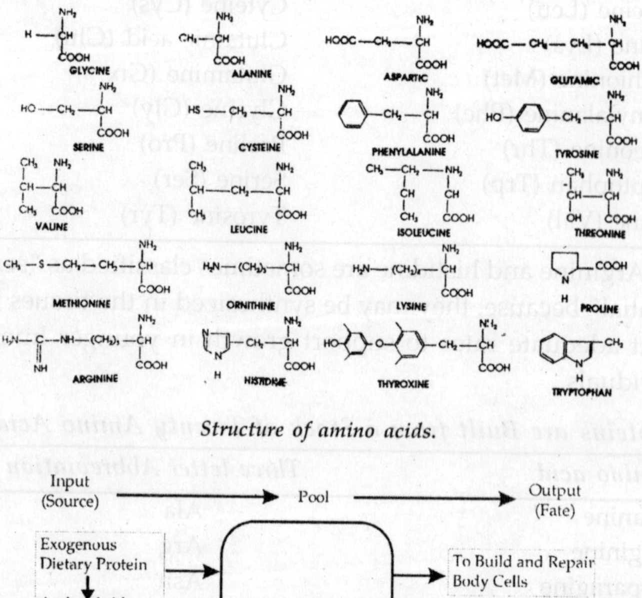

Structure of amino acids.

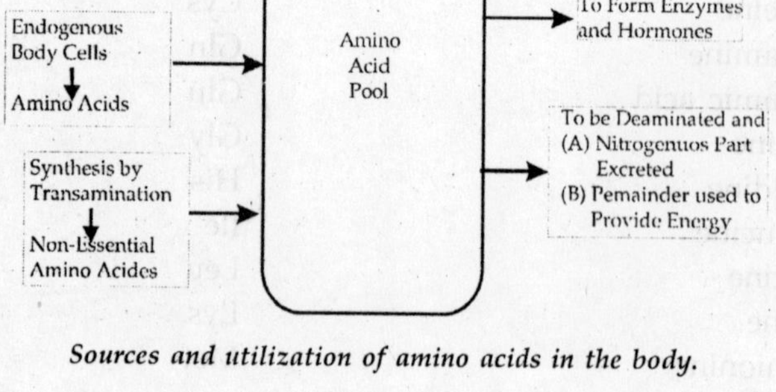

Sources and utilization of amino acids in the body.

Peptides

A peptide consists of two or more amino acids linked by peptide bonds. A peptide may be classified according to the number of amino acid units as a *dipeptide* (2 amino acids), *tripeptide* (3 amino acids) etc. Larger chains composed of many acids are called *polypeptides.* In 1902, Hofmeister and Emil Fischer proposed that the main type of linkage between the amino acids in proteins is the *peptide bond* (also called an *amide bond).* An amino acid unit in a polypeptide is called a residue.

A polypeptide chain consists of a regularly repeating part, called the *backbone* or *main chain,* and a variable part, the distintive *side chains.*

Polypeptides and simple proteins consist entirely of long chain of amino acids linked together by peptide bonds formed between the carboxyl group of one amino acid and the amino group of one amino acid and the amino group of another (CO—NH). A molecule of water is removed during formation of a peptide bond.

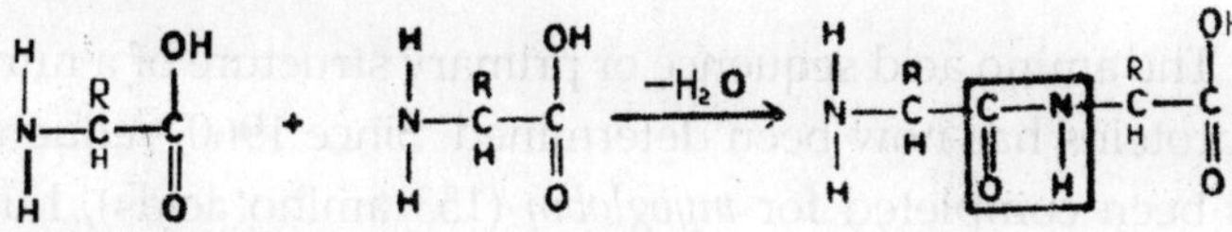

Although the term polypeptide thus should include proteins, polymers consisting of less than 100 amino acid units are arbitrarily termed polypeptides and those with more than 100 are generally termed proteins.

Orders of Protein Structure (Conformation) : The critical determination of the biological function of a protein is its *conformation* which is defined as the three-dimensional arrangement of the atoms of a molecule. Four basic structural, levels are assigned to proteins : primary, secondary, tertiary and quaternary structures :

Primary Structure : The primary structure of a protein refers to the linear sequence of amino acids in the polypeptide chains and location of disulphide bridges, if there are any. The amino acids are linked with each other by peptide bonds only. The primary structure is thus a complete description of the covalent connections of a protein. In 1953 Frederick Sanger elucidated the primary structure of the protein hormone *insulin* (two chains, 21 and 30 amino acids respectively).

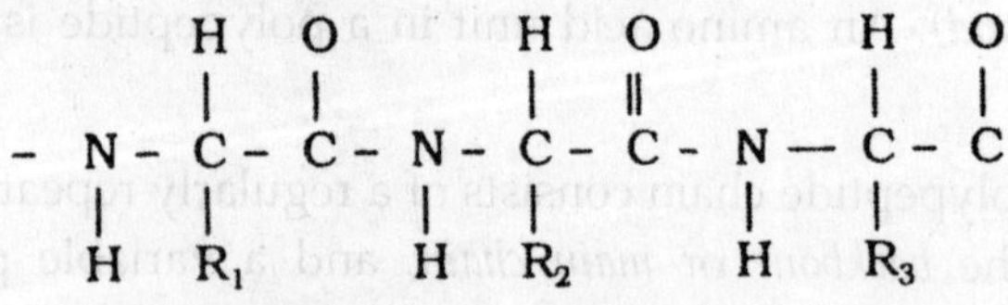

A polypeptide chain is made up of a regularly repeating backbone and distinctive side chains (R_1, R_2, R_3).

Proteins with different activities have widely different primary structures, whereas those having similar roles such as haemoglobin from different species of animals, have similar sequences usually varying by only a few residues in a particular region.

The amino acid sequence or primary structure of a number of proteins has now been determined. Since 1960, sequencing has been completed for *myoglobin* (153 amino acids), human *haemoglobin* (two chains, 141 and 146 amino acid residues respectively), *tobacco mosaic virus protein* (158 residues), and several enzymes such as *ribonuclease (124 residues), cytochrome* C (104—residues), *chymotrypsinogen* (246 residues), and *lysozyme* (129 residues).

Secondary Structure : The folding of a linear polypeptides chain into a specific coiled structure is referred to as the secondary structure of the protein. Such coiling or folding is produced or maintained by hydrogen bonds. The importance of such folding lies in the fact that amino acid residues which may lie far apart in their primary sequence are thereby brought together in close proximity by secondary fonding.

In 1951, Linus Pauling and Robert Corey proposed two periodic polypeptide structures, called the α *-helix* and the β *pleated sheat.*

The Alpha Helix

(a) It is a rod-like structure. The tightly coiled polypeptide main chain forms the inner part of the rod, and the side chains extend outward in a helical manner.

(b) The α helix is stabilized by the hydrogen bonds between the NH and CO groups of the main chain,

(c) The CO group of the each amino acid is hydrogen bonded to the NH group of the amino acid that is situated four residues ahead in the linear sequence. Thus, all the main chain CO and NH groups are hydrogen bonded,

(d) The α helix is a right-handed coil and the hydrogen bonds are parallel to the axis of the helix,

(e) Each residue is related to the next one by a translation of 1.5 Å along the helix axis.

Helical structure is found in *keratin* of hair. The discovery of the structure of the α helix of proteins is considered a major advance in protein chemistry and serves to explain the fibrous structure of many proteins.

The β pleated Sheat : It was the second periodic structural motif elucidated by Pauling and Corey in 1951, the α helix having been the first :

(a) The β pleated sheet differs from the α helix in that it is a *sheat* rather than a *rod.* Here the polypeptide chain is almost fully extended rather than being tightly coiled as in the a helix,

(b) The β pleated sheet is stabilized by hydrogen bonds between NH and CO groups in *different* polypeptide chains, whereas in the a helix the hydrogen bonds are between NH and CO groups in the *same* polypeptide chain.

(c) The axial distance between adjacent amino acids is 3.5 Å, in contrast with 1.5 A for the α helix,

(d) Adjacent chains in a β pleated sheat can run in the same direction *(parallel β sheai)* or in opposite directions *(antiparallel β sheat), e.g.,* silk fibroin

(e) Formation of a β sheet by a single polypeptide chain can occur if the chain folds back on itself. In this state, a loop, connecting antiparallel H-bonded strands in the β conformation, is called a β *turn.* The importance of such folding lies in the fact that amino acid residues which may lie far apart in their primary sequence are thereby brought together in close proximity by secondary fonding.

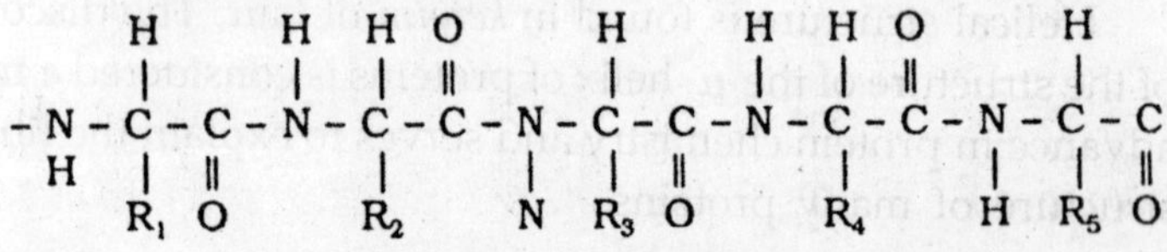

The secondary structure of protein. In the a helix, the CO group of residue n is hydrogen bonded to the NH group of residue (n + 4).

Hydrogen Bonds : In 1936, Mirsky and Pauling suggested that a major factor in maintaining the folded structure of the peptide chain is the presence of hydrogen bonds. The formation of a hydrogen bond is due to the tendency of a hydrogen atom to share the electrons of an oxygen atom. For example, the carbonyl oxygen of one peptide bond shares its electrons with the hydrogen atom of another peptide bond.

C : : O : H : N

Although individual hydrogen bonds of this type are relatively weak as compared with covalent bonds, they will reinforce each other if a molecule contains many such bonds.

Hydrogen bonds can be broken by many physical and chemical treatments, for example, by excessive heat, pressure, pH, electricity, heavy metals and other agents that change the environment of a protein.

The Collagen Helix : (a) It is a third periodic structure responsible for the high tensile strength of collagen, the major protein of skin, bone, and tendon, (b) The basic structural unit of collagan is *tropocollagen* which consists of three polypeptide chains, (c) Each of the three polypeptide chains is in a helical conformation, (d) The three helical strands wind around each other to form a super helical stiff cable or helical rod 3000 Å long and 15 Å in diameter. It is one of the longest known proteins, (e) The three strands are hydrogen bonded to each other. The direction of the hydrogen bond is perpendicular to the long axis of the tropocollagen rod (f) Collagen is unusually rich in glycine and proline and contains hydroxyproline and hydroxylysine, which are found in very few other proteins.

The strength of a collagen fibre is remarkable : a load of at least 10 kg is needed to break a fibre 1 mm in diameter.

Tertiary Structure

The arrangement and inter-relationship of the twisted chains of protein into specific, loops and bends is called the tertiary structure of the protein. Tertiary structure describes how the chains with secondary structure further interact through the R groups of the amino acid residues to a give 3-

Dimensional shape. In other words, interactions between different regions of the secondary chain produce tertiary structure. Tertiary structure is maintained by strong covalent bonds *[Peptide* and *Disulphide bonds)* and weak non-covalent bonds *(Hydrogen bonds, Hydrophobic bonds, Ionic bonds* and *Van der Waal's forces].*

(i) *Hydrogen Bonds* : In this case, these link together relatively far apart portions of a polypeptide chain.

(ii) *Hydrophobic Bonds* : The nonpolar side chains of neutral amino acids tend to be closely associated with one another in proteins. In most globular proteins, at least half of the amino acids have hydro-phobic side chains, which are internally clustered in the folded protein, while hydrophilic polar side chains are external. Water is excluded from the interior of the protein molecule, and the interaction between non-polar groups is called *hydrophobia bonding*. The relationship is non-stoichiometric ; hence no true bond may be said to exist. Nevertheless, these interactions play a significant role in maintaining protein structure.

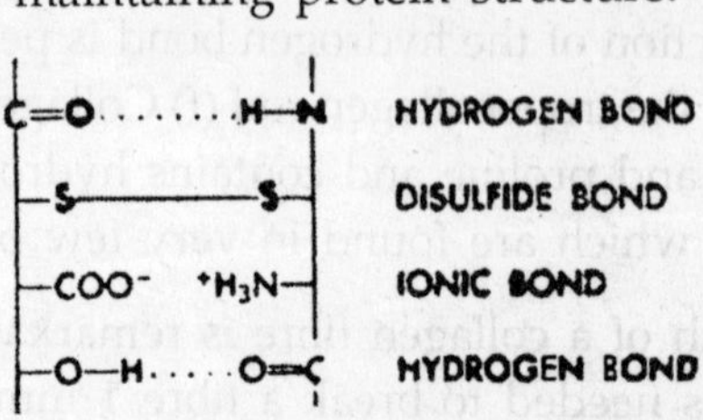

Bonds in Tertiary protien

(iii) *Ionic or Electrostatic Bonds* : These are salt bonds formed between oppositely charged groups in the side chains of amino acids. Some of the amino-acid side chains manifest acid proteins (aspartic acid, glutamic acid), while other manifest the properties of a base (Iysine arginine). When these groups are proximal to one another, they undergo a neutralization reaction, leading to the formation of an ionic bond between them. These bonds have greater energy than the previously discussed linkages, and therefore, tend to be more stable.

(iv) *Disulphide Bonds :* The disulphide bond may interconnect 2 parallel chains through cysteine residues within each polypeptide. A disulphide bridge (- S - S) is formed from the sulphydryl groups (- SH) of two cysteine residues. The resulting disulphide is called cystine. This bond is relatively stable and thus is not readily broken under the usual conditions of denaturation. The polypeptide hormone *insulin* is an excellent examples of the binding together of two peptide chains by disulphide bonds.

Tertiary structure is found in larger proteins like *myoglobin* of muscles and various enzymes. Thermodynamically, this is the most stable structure because enzymatic properties of protein depend on it.

Quaternary Structure

Proteins are said to possess quaternary structure if they consist of 2 or more polypeptide chains united by forces other than covalent bonds *i. e.,* not peptide or disulphide bonds). The forces that stabilize these aggregates are hydrogen bonds and electrostatic or salt bonds formed between amino acids on the polypeptide chains.

A protein with a quaternary structure is composed of several subunits or *monomers.* Such a protein is an *oligomeric* protein. *Dimers* are associations of 2 subunits; *tetramers* are associations of 4 sub units.

Haemoglobin, the oxygen-transporting protein blood, is an excellent example of quaternary structure. This protein consists of four peptide chains of two types : α and β chains that occur in pairs.

Classification of Proteins

The classification of proteins is based upon three general properties, *viz., chemical composition, shape* and *solubility.*

Simple Proteins : Simple proteins consist solely of amino acids.

Fibrous Proteins (Scleroproteins) : These insoluble animal proteins, highly resistant to digestion by proteolytic enzymes, are elongated molecules that may be constituted of several coiled peptide chains that are tightly linked. This group includes the proteins of silk, wool, skin, hair, horn, nails, hoofs, quills, connective tissue and bone. This heterogeneous group may be subdivided into several distinct types :

(1) *Collagens,* the major proteins of connective tissue, are of mesenchymal origin. They are insoluble in water and resistant to animal digestive enzymes, but are altered to easily digestible, soluble *gelatins* by boiling in water, dilute acids or alkalies. Approximately 30% of the total protein in the mammalian body is collagen.

(2) *Ekistins* are present in tendon, arteries and other elastic tissue. Derived from mesenchyme, they cannot be converted to gelatins.

(3) *Keratins* are the proteins of hair, wool, quills, hoofs, nails etc. They are derived from ectoderm.

(4) *Myosin,* the major protein of muscle, is also fibrous protein.

(5) *Ossein* is found in bones and teeth.

Globular Proteins : These are spherical or ovoid in shape because of the presence of peptide chains which are folded or coiled in a very compact manner. They are generally soluble in water or in aqueous media containing salts, acids, bases or alcohol. This group includes enzymes, oxygen-carrying proteins and protein hormones like ACTH, oxytocin, vasopressin, glucagon and insulin. A number of descriptive terms that categorise certain proteins, based on the solubility, are in common use.

(1) *Albumins* are readily soluble in water and coagulable by heat. This is a large group, of which egg white (ovalbumin) and serum albumin are examples. Albumins may be precipitated from solution at high concentrations, a process called "salting out".

(2) *Globulins* are insoluble or sparingly soluble in water, but their solubility is greatly increased by the addition of neutral salts such as NaCl. These proteins are coagulable by heat. Examples are serum globulin, fibrinogen, myosin of muscle and other tissues, ovoglobulin in egg-yolk and globulins (edestin) of plant seeds like squash, soyabean, hemp etc.

(3) *Histones* are basic proteins that are soluble in water and that yield, on hydrolysis, large amounts of arginine or lysine. Histones can be extracted in large amounts from certain glandular tissues, such as thymus and pancrease. Histones are combined with nucleic acids within cells. The globin present in haemoglobin is a histone.

(4) *Protamines* are strongly basic proteins of relatively low molecular weight. They are associated with nucleic acids and are obtained in large quantity from ripe sperm cells of fish, *e.g.*, *salmin* from Salmon sperm, *clupeine* from Herring, and *sturin* from Sturgeon. They contain no sulphur and have a high nitrogen content (25 to 30%) because of the presence of large quantities of arginine.

(5) *Glutelins* are insoluble in distilled water or alcohol but soluble in dilute acid or base solutions. They are commonly found in various plant seeds. Examples are glutenin from wheat and oryzenin from rice.

(6) *Prolamines* are insoluble in absolute alcohol and water but soluble in 70 to 80% alcohol. They may be isolated from various plant seeds ; *e.g.*, zein from maize and gliadin from wheat.

Conjugated Proteins

Conjugated proteins are complex proteins in which the protein molecule is combined with characteristic non-amino acid substances. The term *prosthetic group* is generally used to designate the non amino acid moiety. These include several types such as :

Nucleoproteins : These are combinations of proteins with nucleic acids. Examples are *ribonucleoproteins* found in ribosomes and *deoxyribonucleo proteins* in chromosomes.

Mucoproteins : The protein components of *mucoids* or *mucoproteins* are combined with large amounts (more than 4%) of carbohydrate, measured as *hexosamine.* Well developed soluble mucoproteins have been obtained from egg white (*ovomucoid* α), *orosomucoid* and *haplogobins* (α_2-globulins) from blood serum and from pregnanediol in human pregnancy urine. Soluble mucoproteins are not readily denatured by heat, nor are they easily precipitated by common protein precipitants like trichloroacetic or picric acids.

Glycoproteins : The term glycoprotein is frequently restricted to those proteins that contain small amounts of carbohydrate, less than 4% hexosamine. This group includes many common albumins and globulins. On the basis of their carbohydrate composition and the linkage of the carbohydrate to the protein, glycoproteins have been differentiated into 3 types :

(i) *Plasma Glycoproteins,* which serve as *immunoglobulins* or *antibodies.* There are three major classes of immuglobulins : IgG, IgA and IgM; other minor classes of immunoglobulins found in human plasma are designated as IgD and IgE.

(ii) *Mucin Glycoproteins* of saliva.

(iii) *Mucopolysaccharides* of cartilage, tendons, skin etc.

The distinction between muco and glycoproteins is arbitrary, and intermediate types exist.

Chromoproteins : These are compounds of protein plus a coloured pigment. Examples are haemoglobin, erythrocruorins, haemocyanin, haemerythrin and others given below :

Haemoglobin is a conjugated tetrameric protein. It consists of a large protein molecule, the *globin* consisting of 4 polypeptide chains (two α and two β chains), to each of which is attached a prosthetic *haem* group.

Erythrocruorins are large haemoglobins found in the blood of many polychaete and oligochaete annelid worms and various mollusks.

Haemocyanin is a blue pigment of copper found in the plasma of some mollusks and Crustacea.

Haemerythrin is present in the blood corpuscles of all sipunculid worms, a few polychaete forms and one branchiopod, Ligula.

Myoglobin of muscles is a chromoprotein containing iron.

Cytochromes, the electron carriers in ETS are iron containing chromoproteins.

Chloroplastin found in thylakoids of chloroplastids contain chlorophyll.

Rhodopsin (visual purple) found in the retina of eye contains vitamin A as non-amino acid moiety.

Lipoproteins : These are water soluble proteins containing lipid, *e.g., phosphatidylglycerides, cholesterol, lipo-vitelline* of egg yolk and *serum lipoproteins.*

Metalloproteins : These are metal-binding proteins e.g., A B_1-globulin, termed *transferrin* is capable of combining with iron, copper and zinc. This protein constitutes approximately 3% of the total plasma protein. The prime function of transferrin is to transport iron.

A blue protein containing 0.34% copper, *cendoplasmin,* specifically binds copper and contains practically all the copper in serum ; it is an α_2-globulin.

Ferritin, a storage protein in animals is a metallo protein of iron.

Ferredoxin found in chloroplasts contains iron.

Carbonic anhydrase of blood is a metalloprotein containing zinc.

Plastocyanin, a constituent of ETS is a metalloprotein of copper.

Flavoproteins : The prosthetic group or flavin component (FMN or FAD) remains permanently attached to the enzyme protein (apoenzyme).

Protein — Flavin $\rightleftarrows$ Protein + Flavin

In fact, the flavin groups are usually only separated from the apoenzyme by acid treatment in the cold, or by boiling. Flavoproteins may consist of a single peptide chain with a single flavin, nucleotide or they may be a large, polymeric protein containing not only several flavin components but also one or two metals, one or two haem groups, and another organic electron carrier, *i. e.,* a miniature electron-transport system on a single protein.

Flavoproteins act as enzymes which catalyze oxidation-reduction reactions, *e.g.* liver *D-amino acid oxidase, sucoinic dehydrogenase, xanthine oxidase, dihydro-lipoyldehydrogenase* etc.

Phosphoproteins : These are proteins united with a phosphoric group, *e.g., casein* of milk and *vttelline* of egg-yolk.

Derived Proteins

Derived Proteins are not present in nature as such. They are obtained as a result of partial hydrolysis of natural proteins. These are of two types :

Primary Derived Proteins: These are same-sized like the parental protein, *e.g., protein, metaprotein,* coagulated egg white.

Secondary Derived Proteins : These are smaller than parental proteins, *e.g., proteoses, peptones, peptides.*

Protein → protean → metaprotein → proteose → peptone → polypeptides → lower peptides → amino acids.

Denaturation of Proteins

The conformation of a protein as it occurs under the particular chemical and physical conditions existing in the cells or tissues of the living organism, is called its *native state.* In this state, the protein is biologically active. The comparatively weak forces responsible for maintaining secondary, tertiary, and quaternary structure of proteins are readily disrupted by a variety of environmental changes with a resulting loss of biological activity. This loss of activity is termed *dehydration.*

Causes of Denaturation : The biological activity of most proteins is destroyed by treatment with strong mineral acid or bases, changes in pH, heat applied at or near 100°C, exposure, to heavy metals (Ag, Pb, Hg), physical agitation or treatment with organic solvents at or above room temperature.

Coagulation : Denatured proteins generally are less soluble, and they often precipitate from solution — a process described as *coagulation. A* common example of a protein denatured by heat is the albumin of egg white.

Significance of Denaturation : This property of proteins is used to advantage in the clinical laboratory. Blood or serum samples to be analyzed for small molecules (*e.g.*, glucose, uric acid, drugs) generally are first treated with certain acids to precipitate most of the protein present. This is removed by centrifugation and the protein-free supernatant liquid is then analyzed.

Biological Significance of Proteins

Structural Components of Cells : Some proteins serve as structural materials or as important components of extracellular fluid (ECF). Examples of structural proteins are *myosin* of muscles, *keratin* of skin and hair in mammals and *collagen* of connective tissue. Carbohydrates, fats, minerals and other cellular components are organized around such structural proteins that form the molecular framework of living material.

Food Stuffs : To some extent, particularly in diabetic conditions proteins undergo glueoneogenesis and are used in cells as food stuffs after getting converted into glucose and glycogen.

Biocatalysts (Enzymes) : The most striking characteristic feature of proteins is their ability to function within living cells as reaction-catalyzing enzymes. Enzymes usually enhance reaction rates by at least a million fold. These catalysts vary greatly in biological activity and properties but have in common the fact that they are all proteins of one kind or another. It has been estimated that about 90% of the total protein within a cell is actually enzyme protein. Life depends on enzymatic acceleration of reactions and "living" therefore, means dependance on enzymatic functional proteins. Thus proteins play the unique role of determining the pattern of chemical transformations in biological systems.

Hormones : Hormones from Pancreatic Islets of Langerhans, Pituitary, Parathyroids and Gastrointestinal mucosa are of peptide nature. Likewise, hormones from the Thyroid and Adrenal Medulla are derivatives of amino acid tyrosine.

Oxygen Carriers : *Haemoglobin,* the respiratory pigment of animals, is a conjugated protein composed of colourless basic protein, the globin, and ferroprotoporphyrin or heam. It has a unique ability to bind O_2 in a loose and easily reversible combination. *Myoglobin,* a related protein, transports oxygen in muscle.

Cytochromes, the electron-transfer agents, are basic proteins with an iron containing group derived from protoporphyrin.

Protention against Diseases : Immunoglobulins of the blood plasma (β and γ-globulins) in mammals and other animals act as *antibodies* that neutralize the harmful effects of such foreign agents as viruses, bacteria and cells from other organisms. They also form basis of blood types.

Growth and Repair : Proteins occupy a key position in general body growth and in the repair of wear and tear of the cells and body as a whole. During metabolic activities, tissue protein break down, the these damaged tissues are repaired with the help of amino acids.

Formation of Rhodopsin : The visual purple, rhodopsin is made up of *retinene,* an aldehyde derivative of vitamin A and a protein *opsin.*

Synthesis of Melanin : Melanin, the pigment of skin, hair and choroid layer of eye is derived from the amino acid tyrosine.

Urea Formation : In ureotelic animals, the amino acids ornithine, citrulline and arginine participate in the formation of urea by a cyclic process.

Mineral Nutrients

The mineral elements present in the animal body may be classified as principal elements (macronutrients) and trace elements.

Principal Mineral Elements (Macronutrients) : There are 7 essential elements : calcium, magnesium, sodium, potassium, phosphorus, sulfur, and chlorine. They constitute 60–80% of all the inorganic material in the body.

Calcium

Sources : Of the common foods, milk and cheese are the richest sources of calcium. Most other foods contribute smaller amounts : Examples are egg-yolk, beans, lentils, nuts, figs, cabbage, turnip greens, cauliflower, and asparagus.

Requirements : Men and women after 18 years of age = 800 mg daily. During II and III trimesters of pregnancy and during lactation = 1.2 g daily.

Infants under 1 year = 350 – 540 mg daily.

Children 1–18 years = 0.8 – 1.2 g daily.

Functions

(1) It is major constituent of bones and teeth. About 99% of the body calcium is in the skeleton, where it is maintained as deposits of calcium phosphates in a soft, fibrous matrix.

(2) Ionized calcium is of great importance in blood coagulation.

(3) It maintains the normal excitability of heart.

(4) It is required for muscle contraction and nerve irritability.

(5) It is important in the differential aspects of membrane permeability.

Deficiency : Calcium deficiency results in poor development of bones, dental disorders, stunted growth, rickets in children and osteoporosis in adults.

Phosphorus

Sources and Requirements : Phosphorus is present in nearly all foods. Since the distribution of calcium and of phosphorus in foods is very similar, an adequate intake of calcium generally ensures an adequate intake also of phosphorus. The average daily intake of phosphorus should be about 1.5 g.

Functions

(1) Phosphorus is found in every cell of the body, but most of it (about 80% of the total) is combined with calcium in the bones and teeth.

(2) It is required for phosphorylation associated with energy yielding metabolic reactions.

Deficiency: Phosphorus deficiency leads to poor mineralization of bones and teeth, rickets, osteomalacia and poor growth.

Magnesium

Sources : Derivates of cocoa, various nuts, soyabeans, and some sea foods are relatively rich in magnesium. Whole grains, raw dried beans and peas contain small amounts.

Requirements : The current recommendation for magnesium in the diet is 350 mg/day for adult men and 300 mg/day for adult women.

Functions

(1) The body contains about 21 g of magnesium 70% is combined with calcium and phosphorus in the complex salts of bone.

(2) Magnesium is one of the principal cations of soft tissue

(3) In muscle and other tissue, intracellular magnesium ions probably functions as activators of the phosphate group transfer enzymes.

Deficiency : Magnesium deficiency in man induces neuromuscular dysfunction as manifested by hyperexcitability with muscle tremor and convulsion.

Sodium

Sources : The main source of sodium is the table salt (sodium chloride) used in cooking and seasoning ; ingested foods contain additional sodium. In addition to salted foods, the content of sodium is high in bread, cheese, clams, oysters, wheat germ, and whole grains. Relatively high in sodium are such foods as carrots, cauliflower, celery, eggs, legumes, milk, nuts, spinach, turnips, prunes and radishes.

Requirements : Daily requirements of 5 to as much as 15 g of sodium chloride have been recommended for adults by various authorities.

Functions

(1) This element is the major component of the cations of the extracellular fluid.

(2) It is largely associated with chloride and bicarbonate in regulation of acid-base equilibrium.

(3) It maintains the osmotic pressure of body fluid and thus protects the body against excessive fluid loss.

(4) It also functions in the preservation of normal irritability of muscle and the permeability of the cells.

Deficiency : Due to high environmental temperature, extreme sweating may cause the loss of considerable sodium in the sweat. This results in muscular cramps of the extremities and abdomen, headaches, nausea, and diarrhoea.

Potassium

Sources and Requirements : A high content of potassium is found in the following foods : veal, chicken, beef liver, beef, pork ; dried apricots, dried peaches, bananas, the juices of oranges, and pineapples ; yams and potatoes.

The normal intake of potassium in food is about 4 g/day. This element is so widely distributed that a deficiency is unlikely except in the pathologic states.

Functions

(1) Potassium is the principal cation of the intracellular fluid : but it is also a very important constituent of the extracellular fluid because it influences muscle activity particularly the cardiac muscle.

(2) Within the cells it regulates acid-base balance and osmotic pressure of the intracellular fluid.

(3) High intracellular potassium concentrations are essential for several important metabolic functions including protein biosynthesis by ribosomes.

(4) A number of enzymes, including the glycolytic enzyme *pyruvate kinase,* require K^+ for maximal activity.

Elevated Serum Potassium (Hyperkalemia) : Toxic elevation of serum potassium is confined for the most part to patients with renal failure, advanced dehydration or shock. The symptoms of hyperkalemia are chiefly cardiac and central nervous system depression.

Low Serum Potassium (Hypokalemia) : Potassium deficiency is likely to develop in chronic wasting diseases with malnutrition, gastrointestinal losses, and in metabolic alkalosis. In most of these cases intracellular potassium is transferred to the extracellular fluid, and this potassium is quickly removed by the kidneys.

The symptoms of low serum potassium concentrations include muscle weakness, irritability and paralysis: tachycardia and dilation of the heart are also noted.

Chlorine

Sources and Requirements : In the diet, the chloride occurs almost entirely as sodium chloride, and therefore the intake of chloride is satisfactory as long as sodium intake is adequate.

Functions

(1) As a component of the sodium chloride, the element chlorine (as chloride ion) is essential in water balance and osmotic pressure regulation.

(2) To maintain the acid-base equilibrium, chloride plays a special role in the blood by the action of chloride shift.

(3) In gastric juice, chloride is also of special importance in the production of hydrochloric acid.

Deficiency : Which loss of sodium are excessive, as in diarrhoea, profuse sweating, and certain endocrine disturbances, chloride deficit is likewise observed.

In loss of gastric juice by vomitting or in pyloric or duodenal obstruction, there is a loss of chloride in excess of sodium. This leads to a decrease in plasma chloride, with a compensatory increase in bicarbonate and a resultant hypochloremic alkalosis.

Sulfur

Sources : The main sources of sulfur for the body are the amino acids *cysteine* and *methionine*. Other organic compounds of sulfur are heparin, glutathione, thiamine, biotin, taurocholic acid and the chondroitin sulfate in cartilage, tendon, and bone matrix. Small amounts of inorganic sulfates ; with sodium and potassium, are present in blood and other tissues.

Functions

(1) Participates in the structure of *insulin* and many other proteins.

(2) Specific sulfhydryl groups of crysteine residues in some enzyme molecules are essential for catalytic activity.

(3) Methionine is the principal methyl group donor in the body. The 'activated' form of methionine. S-adenosyl-methionine, functions as a precursor in the synthesis of a large number of methylated compounds involved in intermediary metabolism and detoxification mechanisms.

Trace Elements

These elements occur in living tissues in small amounts. They are classified (roughly in order of importance) as follows:

(1) *Essential Trace Elements (micronutrients)* : Iron, iodine, copper, zinc, manganese, cobalt, molybdenum, selenium, chromium and flourine.

(2) *Possibly Essential Trace Elements* : Nickle, tin, vanadium and silicon.

(3) *Nonessential Trace Elements* : Aluminium, boron, germanium, cadmium, arsenic, lead, and mercury.

Iron

Sources : The best dietary sources of iron are "organ meats" : liver, heart, kidney and spleen. Other good sources are egg-yolk, whole wheat, fish, oysters, clams, nuts, dates, figs, beans, spinach and molasses.

Requirements : The need for iron in the human diet varies greatly at different ages and under different circumstances. It is determined by the requirements for tissue growth and haemoglobin synthesis and the replacement needs due to iron losses in urine, faeces, and in the female, the additional losses in menstruation , gestation and lactation. The need for iron is greatest during the first 2 years of life, during the period of rapid growth and haemoglobin increase in adolescence, and throughout the childbearing period in women.

The recommended daily amounts of iron currently suggested by nutritional authorities are as follows :

A. Infants : 10 – 15 mg.

B. Children : 1 – 3 years of age, 15 mg ; 4 – 10 years of age, 10 mg.

C. Older Children and Adults : *Males* .11–18 years of age, 18 mg ; after 19 years of age, 10 mg. *Females* : 11–50 years of age, and during pregnancy or lactation 18 mg. After 51 years of age, 10 mg.

Functions

(1) The role of iron in the body is almost exclusively confined to the processes of cellular respiration. Iron porphyrin (haeme) groups are essential components of *haemoglobin, myoglobin,* the *cytochromes,* and the enzymes *catalase* and *peroxidase.*

(2) Nonhaem iron is almost entirely protein bound. These forms include the intracellular iron-containing flavoproteins (NADH dehydrogenase) and iron-sulfur proteins as well as storage and transport forms of the mineral.

Iron Deficiency : Iron deficiency anemias are of the *hypochromic microcytic* type. A deficiency or iron may result from inadequate intake or inadequate absorption as well as from excessive loss of blood. Deficiency of iron causes the bone-marrows to produce small cells (microcytic) with less than optimum haemoglobin content (hypochromic).

In severe iron deficiency, the rate of RBC formation is curtailed causing a low red cell count. Symptoms of the disease include a pale skin, loss of appetite, low energy, easy fatigue, palpitation and shortness of breath. The disease can be cured by giving drugs containing ferrous salts.

Copper

Sources : The richest sources of dietary copper are nuts, some shellfish, liver, kidney, raisins and dried legumes. Cow's milk is a poor source of copper.

Requirements : A daily allowance of 2.5 mg is sufficient for adults ; infants and children require about 0.05 mg/kg body weight.

Functions

(1) Copper is an essential constituent of several proteins, metalloenzymes, and some naturally occurring pigments.

(2) It is essential for haemoglobin synthesis, normal bone formation, and the maintenance of myelin within the nervous system.

(3) Haemocyanin is a copper-protein complex in the blood of certain invertebrates, where it functions like haemoglobin as an oxygen carrier.

(4) Copper is present in the most important enzyme of aerobic metabolism: *Cytochrome C oxidase,* which is responsible for the major part of the oxygen consumed by life on this planet.

Deficiency : A nutritional deficiency of copper has never been positively demonstrated in man, although it has been suspected in cases of sprue or in nephrosis. However, there are reports of a syndrome in infants which is characterized by low levels of serum copper and iron and by oedema and a hypochromic microcytic anemia.

Iodine

Sources and Requirements : It is found in traces as iodides in water, food and common salts. Sea-food and iodized salts are the best sources.

The requirements for iodine is 5 μ g/100 cal or, for adults, about 100–150 μ g/day. The use of iodized salt regularly will provide more than this.

Functions : Iodine is required exclusively for the biosynthesis of the iodinated thyroid hormones : Tri-iodothyronine (T_3 and Tetra-iodothyronine (T_4).

Deficiency : Iodine deficiency results in thyroid hypertrophy.

Manganese

Sources and Requirements : Nuts and whole grains are rich sources of manganese ; vegetables and fruits are good sources. Meats, poultry, seafoods, and fish are poor sources.

An evident deficiency of manganese is not known in man, suggesting that the average daily dietary intake of 2.5–7 mg is adequate.

Functions

(1) Manganese is essential for normal bone structure, reproduction, and the normal functioning of the central nervous system.

(2) The enzyme *pyruvate carboxylase,* involved in gluconeogenesis contains tightly bound manganese.

(3) Arginase is specifically activated by manganese ions.

(4) In human serum, manganese is bound to a specific β-globulin.

Cobalt

This element is a constituents of vitamin B_{12}, which is necessary for normal red blood cell formation. Enzymes requiring vitamin B_{12} for activity include *methyl-malonyl CoA mutase, methyl tetrahydrofolate oxidoreductase, homocysteine, methyltransferase* and *ribonucleotide reductase.*

Cobalt is widely distributed throughout the body. The highest concentrations are usually found in the liver, kidneys and bones.

Zinc

Sources and Requirements : A balanced diet containing sufficient animal protein should provide the adequate daily zinc requirement. Meat, liver, eggs, seafood, milk, and whole grain products are good sources.

The currently recommended allowance is 15 mg/day for adults, with an additional 15 mg during pregnancy and 10 mg during location.

Functions

(1) Zinc is essential for the normal growth, reproduction, and life expectancy of animals.

(2) It has a beneficial effect on the processes of tissue repair and wound healing.

(3) The element is an essential component of a number of enzymes present in animal tissue, including *alcohol dehydrogenase, alkaline phosphatase, carbonic anhydrase, procarboxypeptidase.*

(4) The retina contains a zinc metalloenzyme, *retinene reductase,* which is required for the reconstitution of retinene (vitamin A aldehyde) during the rhodopsin cycle.

(5) Zinc is necessary to maintain normal concentrations of vitamin A in plasma.

(6) Insulin forms complexes with zinc. Zinc adhering to the insulin molecule increases the duration of insulin action when given by injection.

Zinc is widely distributed in the tissues of the body. About 20% of the total body zinc is present in the skin. A considerable proportion is also present in the bones and teeth. High concentration of zinc are found in spermatozoa, prostrate, and epididymis.

Deficiency : Pronounced zinc deficiency in man, resulting in hypogonadism and dwarfism, has been found in the middle East.

Flourine

Sources and Requirements : Drinking water is the main source of flouride of humans. At a concentration of 1 ppm, flouride is supplied in nutritionally adequate amounts. When the drinking water in a given area contains less than that amount, it is regarded as an excellent public health practice to add flouride to the water supply (fluoridation) in order to raise its concentration to an appropriate level.

Functions

(1) The protective effect of fluoride in tooth development is most important during infancy and early childhood. It prevent dental caries.

(2) Appropriate levels of dietary fluoride decrease the incidence of osteoporosis.

Fluorosis

In excessively high intake of fluoride during childhood causes mottling and discolouration of the enamel of the teeth. Intake of fluoride in very large quantities also causes changes in bone, including increased bone density, and calcification at the point of insertion of muscles. Fluorosis occurs only in geographic areas where the water naturally contains unusually high concentrations of fluoride (as much as 10–45 ppm) : it does not occur in communities with properly controlled system for fluoridation of the water supply.

The Role of Minerals in Human Nutrition

S. No.	Name	Functions	Important Sources	Effects of Deficiency
1.	Calcium	Most abundant mineral-element in the body required for muscle contraction, normal heart rhythm and nerve irritability. Major constituent of bones and teeth.	Milk, cheese, eggs yolk, beans, nuts. cabbage, turnip, shrimps.	Poor development of bones, dental disorders, stunted growth, rickets in children; may contribute to osteoporosis in adults,
2.	Iron	Constituent of Haemoglobin, myoglobin and some oxidative enzymes.	Liver, heart, kidney and spleen are best sources. Other good sources are egg-yolk, nuts, dates, figs, beans, spinach and molasses.	Reduced haemoglobin level and anemia,
3.	Sodium	Participates in the regulation of muscle and nerve irritability. Regulates osmotic pressure of the extra-cellular fluids. Buffer salts.	Table salt, meat, fish, milk, eggs and sodium compounds like baking soda and baking powder,	Nausea; muscular cramps. diarrhoea. dehydration,

Contd...

S. No.	Name	Functions	Important Sources	Effects of Deficiency
4.	Potassium	Participates in the regulation of muscle and nerve irritability and affects heart rhythm. Regulates osmotic pressure of intracellular fluid.	Meat, fish cereals, dried apricots, bananas, juice of oranges and pineapples and potatoes,	Nervous disorders, poor muscular control and slow heart rate.
5.	Chlorine	In association with sodium and potassium, chlorine conri-butes to maintain normal body water content. It is a constituent of gastric juice and maintains acid-base balance.	Table salt, milk, meat, eggs.	Continued vomitting may lead to deficiency followed by alkalosis.
6.	Phosphorus	Major constituent of bones and teeth-. Required for phosphory-lation associated with energy-yielding metabolic reactions. Buffer salt.	Milk, cheese, meat, egg-yolk, pulses, nuts and cereals.	Poor mineralization of bones and teeth rickets, osteomalacia, poor growth.

Contd...

S. No.	Name	Functions	Important Sources	Effects of Deficiency
7.	Iodine	Constituent of thyroid hormones	In traces as iodides in water. food and common salts. Sea-foods and Iodized salt.	Nutritional deficiency may produce simple goitre, low BMR and nervous disorders.
8.	Copper	Required in haemoglobin synthesis, constituent of enzymes like cytochrome oxidase. catalase, uricase, oxidase etc.	Legumes, whole-grain cereals, nuts, liver, meat, fish, etc.	Anemia in infants.
9.	Magnesium	Constituent of teeth, bones and many other tissues. Affects muscle and nerve function. Acts on sonie enzymes of glycolysis.	Cereals nuts, legumes. cocoa meat and milk.	Dietary deficiency not known in man.
10.	Sulfur	Constituent of keratin of hair, Insulin and many proteins.	Eggs, cheese, milk, meat, nuts and pulses.	

Molybdenum

Functions and Distribution : Molybdenum is an essential component of the molybdoflavoproteins *xanthine oxidase* and *aldehyde oxidase* and the molybdohaemo protein *sulfite oxidase* of animal tissues.

Molybdenum concentrations in animal tissues are normally very low. The highest concentrations of molybdenum are usually found in liver and kidney.

2

Nutrition Mechanism

Food as Source of Energy

All the living animals require food for three main purposes which are as follows:

1. For movements, and muscle contraction,
2. For growth and synthesis of body substances, and
3. As a fuel to supply energy and materials for maintenance.

Thus *food* may be defined as any substance that, when taken into the body, will furnish energy and materials for the structure and repair of tissues.

Modes of Nutrition

There are many approaches to classifying the ways in which organisms obtain their food. A common approach is to divide organisms into *autotrophs* and *heterotrophs.*

Autotrophic Nutrition : Autotrophs are organisms that literally 'feed themselves'. Green plants are the most obvious autotrophs. They need only visible light, water, carbon dioxide and inorganic ions to survive, grow and reproduce. The process of photosynthesis enables them to synthesize all the complex organic molecules, that they require from these simple building blocks. Because these organisms use light as their energy source, they are called *photoautotrophs.*

However, some micro-organisms are *chemoautotrophs.* They obtain their energy not from sunlight but from certain specific chemical reactions involving only inorganic substrates. They are also called *chemosynthetic organisms.*

Heterotrophic Nutrition : Organisms that cannot synthesize their own food are called heterotrophs. Animals are the most obvious heterotrophs. They need to take in an external source of organic carbon. While autotrophs such as green plants and chemosynthetic bacteria obtain the few nutrients that they require from their environment, *heterotrophs* have first to *ingest* their food. Their food is then digested, absorbed, and assimilated and finally some matter is egested.

Heterotrophs differ greatly in the kinds of food they ingest and in the ways they obtain their food. Three main types of heterotrophic nutrition are commonly recognised. These are *holozoic nutrition* (animals feeding on relatively large pieces of dead organic material), *parasitic nutrition* (animals obtaining their food from their host), and *saprotrophic nutrition* (organisms feeding on dead organic matter which they either absorb in solution or ingest as very small pieces). Most saprotrophs obtain their food by extracellular digestion in which enzymes are secreted on to the food source and the soluble products are then absorbed. This is the technique used by bacteria, fungi and housefly for instance.

All the food requirements of animals are satisfied by the intake of organic materials of plant or animal origin. The common *classification of food* includes carbohydrates, proteins, fats, water, minerals, salts and vitamins. The first three are required for energy and building of materials, the latter three for building and regulative action.

Although the needs of all animals for these substances are almost similar, they have different ways and means of getting them. Some animals are exclusively *herbivorous* (rabbit), others are exclusively *carnivorous* (tiger) and still others are *omnivorous* (man). There are also differences in the amount and kind of food required. For example, rats do not need ascorbic acid, since they make this vitamin in their own body. But man must include it in his diet. Water is acquired by animals in different ways. Aquatic animals take in large amounts with their food, frogs through their skin and some forms make use of the water formed in the oxidation of their food. Some herbivores may have an intense liking for salt, but carnivores usually dislike it.

Balanced Diet

Balanced diet is one of the basic concepts of nutrition. The diet or food intake may be considered under two general headings.

(i) the nutritionally adequate, or *balanced diet* and

(ii) special diets prescribed for treatment or prevention of disease states—for example, the low calorie diet prescribed for obesity.

A nutritionally adequate or *balanced diet* contains necessary amounts of the six essentials of human nutrition : proteins, carbohydrates, fats, vitamins, minerals and water.

Many systems for assuming a *balanced diet* have been worked out. A comparatively simple and convenient one was worked out during World War II, and has been generally accepted under the name of the *'Basic 7'*. This system of food selection assures an adequate supply of protective foods daily. *Choose one food daily from each of the following groups :*

Group 1 : leafy, green and yellow vegetables.

Group 2 : citrus fruits, tomatoes, raw cabbage.

Group 3 : potatoes and other vegetables and fruits (select 2 items from this group).

Group 4 : milk and milk products.

Group 5 : meat, poultry, fish, eggs, nuts.

Group 6 : bread, flour, and cereals.

Group 7 : butter and fortified margarine.

According to a report four well defined food groups are : milk products (group I), meat products (group II), vegetables and fruits (group III), and cereal grain foods (group IV). Therefore, for a balanced diet foods from all the four groups should be commonly consumed by each person each day.

Caloric Requirements in Diet : An immense amount of scientific research has gone into the subject of human nutrition and it has been found out that food requirements and *caloric needs* differ with age, sex, body size and weight, pregnancy and climate. Occupation and physical activity may also change dietary needs. The quantity of Calories needed to maintain an individual is generally no less than 2250 and usually not more than 3000 per day (This unit is not to be confused with the small calorie, or "calorie"; it is called large calorie, kilocalorie or Calorie; it is the amount of released heat which raises the temperature of 1 kilogram of water from 15° to 16° Centigrade).

According to FAO report (1957), a man of 25 years, weighing 65 kg, would require 3200 Calories per day, while a woman of 25 years, weighing 55 kg, needs only 2300 Calories per day. The calorie intake of growing children is more as it must allow for growth and physical development. Calorie requirements for various activities differ considerably. For example, sleeping requires only 60 Calories per hour; other activities such as driving, standing, brisk walking and swimming require 90,150,180 and 270 Calories per hour respectively *(Bernarde, 1968)*.

Malnutrition and Nutritional Diseases : A deviation from balanced nutrition (undernutrition of one or more elements of diet, overnutrition, etc.) is termed malnutrition. It means insufficient and faulty nutrition. In some cases morphological and physiological symptoms of malnourishment are severe. As a result, several *nutritional-deficiency diseases* are caused, some of which are as follows:

Goitre is one of the principal diseases that are caused by inadequate nutrition. If the intake of iodine is insufficient, the thyroid gland enlarges in its attempt to supply adequate combined iodine to the body. In severe cases, however, cretinism and thyroid cancer may occur. The addition of iodine to salt prevents the widespread occurrence of goitre.

Hypochromic anaemia is a disease which is the result of inadequate intake of iron. As a result, haemoglobin of the blood is reduced and the red blood cells appear pale or hypochromic.

Diseases of the eye, such as nyctalopia, night blindness, xerophthalmia, loss of sight due to prolonged dryness of cornea are diseases that result from deficiency of vitamin A.

Rickets, a disease of children, results from the lack of vitamin D. Deficiency of vitamin D in adults produces "adult rickets" or osteomalacia.

Severe deficiency of one of the B-complex vitamins, thiamine, produces *beri-beri*. It is characterised by gastro-intestinal problems, muscular weakness, paralysis of feet and legs, enlarged heart, and emaciation. A diet of polished rice is the most common cause of the disease, because the thiamine exists in the outer brown layer of the grain, which is removed during polishing.

Inadequate quantities of riboflavin, the yellow B-complex vitamin, causes *ariboflavinosis*. Symptoms of the disease include morphological changes in the tongue and lips and impairment of vision.

The deficiency of B-vitamin, niacin, is believed to cause *pellagra*. Late symptoms of the disease include a characteristic dermatitis in which the skin becomes cracked, red and scaly.

Extreme protein deficiency during malnutrition causes the disease called *kwashiorkor*. Symptoms include lack of growth, retarded development, high levels of growth hormone, apathy, lack of appetite, diarrhoea, edema, and changes in the hair texture and colour. The disease is treated by feeding reconstituted non-fat dry milk or vegetable protein concoctions.

It has been shown that under severe conditions of protein malnutrition, adequate calories alone are not sufficient to correct the excess secretion of growth hormone. Instead, the protein deficiency must also be corrected before the growth hormone concentration will return to normal.

Inadequate proteins and calories in the diet cause *marasmus* (also called *sukha* or "drying up"). Marasmus is quite common in village children in India. It is characterized by wizened, shrunken features, and sluggish matchstick extremities. These babies also suffer from diarrhoea and respiratory infections.

Besides the physical debility associated with malnutrition, poor mental development is also known. Unfortunataly, the acute effects of malnutrition occur at the time when the child's brain is developing fastest. Experiments on dogs and other animals have also shown physical and behavioural effects of malnutrition. In extreme cases of malnutrition death may occur.

Chemical Nature and other Properties of the Food Components

1. *Carbohydrates* : The term carbohydrate stems from the fact that many of the sugars have the empirical formula $C_nH_{2n}O_n$, which corresponds technically to a *'hydrate of carbon'*. Thus, *"carbohydrates are compounds of carbon, hydrogen and oxygen, derived more or less directly from CO_2 and H_2O in photosynthesis"*. A carbohydrate is chemically defined as an organic compound that contains a carbonyl group (aldehyde or ketone) in addition to two or more alcohol groups, or that yields such compounds upon hydrolysis. Sugar, starch and cellulose are examples of carbohydrates. Structurally, they are usually classified as *monosaccharides (e.g.,* glucose, fructose, ribose and deoxyribose), *disaccharides (e.g.,* lactose, sucrose), and *polysaccharides (e.g.,* starch and cellulose).
2. *Proteins* : The term protein is derived from the Greek word *proteios,* meaning *of the first rank",* for proteins occupy a central position in the structural and functional characteristics of the living beings. Proteins may be defined, in chemical sense, as *"high-molecular-weight polymers in which the building blocks are the amino acids"*. Polymers made up of small number of amino acids (2, 3, 4, to about 100) are commonly called *peptides* or *polypeptides,* whereas those formed of a large number of units (upto 10,000 or more) are called proteins. They are generally classified as *simple proteins (e.g.,* albumins, globulins, etc.) and *conjugated proteins (e.g.,* nucleoproteins, mucoproteins, glycoproteins, etc.). Upon hydrolysis, simple proteins are isolated into different amino acids, whereas conjugated proteins upon hydrolysis yield non-amino acid components as well as amino acids.
3. *Fats* : Fats *and oils are esters of the alcohol glycerol and various high-molecular-weight carboxylic acids* (also called

fatty acids). Esters of this type are usually referred to as *glycerides.* Thus, most common fats are complex mixtures of glycerides containing several different fatty acids. Upon hydrolysis they yield fatty acids and an alcohol. In the formula of a fat

$$\begin{array}{l} R\text{—COO—}CH_2 \\ \qquad\qquad\quad | \\ R'\text{—COO—}CH \\ \qquad\qquad\quad | \\ R''\text{—COO—}CH_2 \end{array}$$

given above, —R, — R′, and R″ represent the long carbon chains of either the same or different fatty acids. The two most common saturated fatty acids found in animal fats are *palmitic* and *stearic* acid. Several unsaturated fatty acids, not synthesized by the body must be provided by the diet and are, therefore, termed as *essential fatty acids.* The glycerides of the unsaturated fatty acids tend to have lower melting points than the glycerides of saturated fatty acids, and most oils are composed of predominantly of glycerides of unsaturated fatty acids.

4. *Water :* Water is chemically, an oxide of hydrogen (H_2O), and is most essential for life. It acts as a medium of transport of food materials and plays other vital roles in cellular physiology. Generally there is a daily loss of about 1500 ml of water by normal human adults. Of this, about 600 ml is lost through the skin in perspiration, 400 ml in the expired air, and 500 ml in the urine. When the intake is less than this obligatory loss of 1500 ml, the difference is met by the total body water. Since the oxidation of glucose and lipid, in an amount sufficient to yield 2000 kcal per day, results in the formation of about 300 ml of water (metabolic water), an intake of 1200 ml per day appears necessary.
5. *Mineral Nutrients :* Minerals play important role in

metabolism and are among the essential food items. The minerals required are sodium chloride for the blood and osmotic balance of the body, iron for the haemoglobin of the blood, potassium and magnesium for muscle contraction, calcium and phosphorus for the teeth and bones, and iodine for the hormone of the thyroid gland. As there is steady loss of these salts from the body, they must be replaced in the food we eat. The chief source of NaCI is table salt, iron — meats and eggs, potassium and magnesium—milk and meat, and iodine — drinking water or ionized table salt. In addition human diets require magnesium, manganese, copper, zinc, molybdenum, and selenium, which serve as cofactors for various enzymes. The zinc deficiency is reflected in lack of growth and in hypogonadism during adolescence. The most severe clinical disorder caused by zinc deficiency is the disease acrodermatitis enteropathica which begins in infancy and is manifested by rough and thick skin, baldness, and persistent diarrea, followed by poor growth, infections and death in a few years.

6. *Vitamins* : The term *"vitamin"* was first introduced in 1912 by *Funk* to designate the special unknown organic nutrients whose deficiency in the diet causes some diseases. Thus, *vitamins are organic compounds which are needed in extremely small quantities in the diet and are essential for the normal functioning of an organism.* The vitamins are generally classified as *fat-soluble vitamins* and *water-soluble vitamins.* In digestion, vitamins act as enzymes.

Fat Soluble Vitamins

These are vitamins A, D, E and K.

Vitamin A : Vitamin A (Fig.) is also known as Axerophthol, Antiophthalmic (or antixerophthalmic) vitamin, and Retinol.

This vitamin includes the compounds that are derivatives of the *carotene* pigments synthesized by plants. Carotene becomes vitamin A by enzymatic hydrolysis :

$$C_{40}H_{56} + 2H_2O \longrightarrow 2C_{20}H_{30}O$$

carotene vitamin A

Thus, in the presence of water one molecule of carotene splits into two molecules of vitamin A.

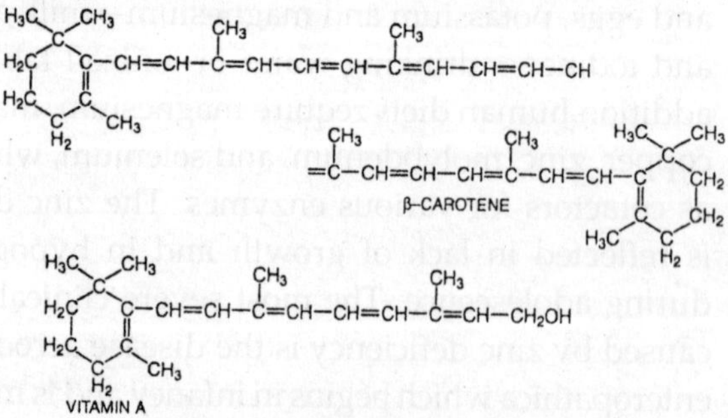

Structure of β-carotene and vitamin A.

Source : Vitamin A is found as such in the fat of milk and in milk products like butter or cream and in the egg. It is found in quite large amounts in liver fat, especially in cod or shark-liver oil. However, green vegetables and carrots do not contain vitamin A, but they have variable amounts of carotene which are provitamins or precursors of vitamin A. The approximate daily requirement of vitamin A is 1.5 mg.

Function : Vitamin A and carotene are absorbed from the small intestine together with fat. Vitamin A has multiple functions and plays a highly important role in vision. Both the rods and cones of the eye contain light-sensitive pigments, which require vitamin A for their formation and functioning. When the eye is exposed to light, rhodopsin or visual purple (pigment of rods) is bleached and two substances, retinol and opsin (a protein) are produced. In the dark, rhodopsin is regenerated and the sensitivity of the eye to light is restored. Thus, the speed of dark-adaptation, *i e.*, the ability to see better in the dark, depends on the speed of reformation of the broken down rhodopsin. If there is insufficient retinol present in the retina, visual purple cannot be restored and *night blindness* results.

The lack of vitamin A also causes *xerophthalmia* (a disease of the eye causing inhibition of lachrymal secretion and drying of the cornea), changes in the skin, and retardation in growth. Vitamin A is essential for the maintenance of epithelial cells of skin. It is also involved in the metabolism of carbohydrates and nucleic acids and may be concerned in the electron transport system. Vitamin A also seems to be involved in the synthesis of mucopolysaccharides, especially chondroitin sulphate. It is also essential for spermatogenesis, and for development and maintenance of placenta.

Vitamin D : Vitamin D is also known as antirachitic vitamin. The principal natural *vitamers* (structurally related compounds possessing qualitatively similar activity) of this vitamin are: Vitamin D_2 (calciferol, ergocalciferol) and vitamin D_3 (cholecalciferol). One international unit of vitamin D is defined as the activity of 0.025 μg of cholecalciferol.

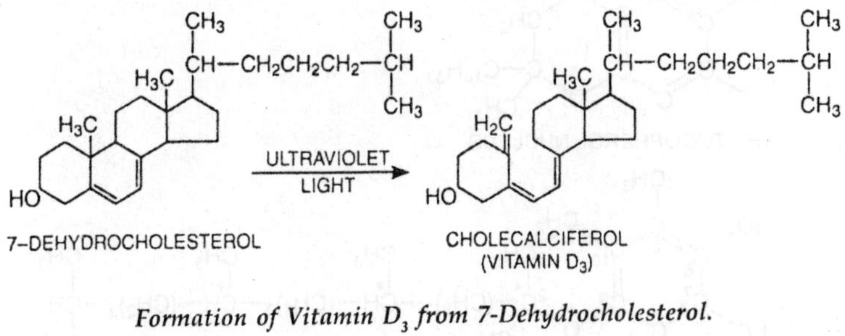

Formation of Vitamin D_3 from 7-Dehydrocholesterol.

Source : Vitamin D is found mainly in fish liver oil and in yolk of egg. It is also present in small amount in beef fat and milk. Vitamin D_2 is formed by ultraviolet irradiation of ergosterol (a substance found in yeast and ergot, from which it is named). Vitamin D_3 occurs naturally in fish-liver oil and egg yolk. It is formed when 7-dehydrocholesterol of the skin is activated by ultraviolet light (Fig.). The approximate daily requirement of vitamin D is 10 μg.

Function : The most important function of vitamin D is that it increases calcium and phosphate absorption from the gut. It also promotes calcification by a direct action on bone. It prevents and cures rickets. Lack of vitamin D prevents the absorption of calcium, which leads to a fall in blood calcium levels and a resultant defect in bone formation (osteomalacia). The action of vitamin D may be compared with that of aldosterone.

Vitamin E : Vitamin E is also called α-tocopherol or antisterility vitamin (Fig.). The discovery of vitamin E in 1932 was based on the experiment of *Evans* who showed that for normal reproductive function rats require a fat-soluble factor present in crude vegetable oils. This factor was later identified as an analogous series called tocopherols (from the Greek for "young-bearing"). Vitamin E was isolated from wheat-germ oil in 1936 and given the name *tocopherol* (Gk. *tokos* = childbirth, *phero* = to bear, *ol* = an alcohol).

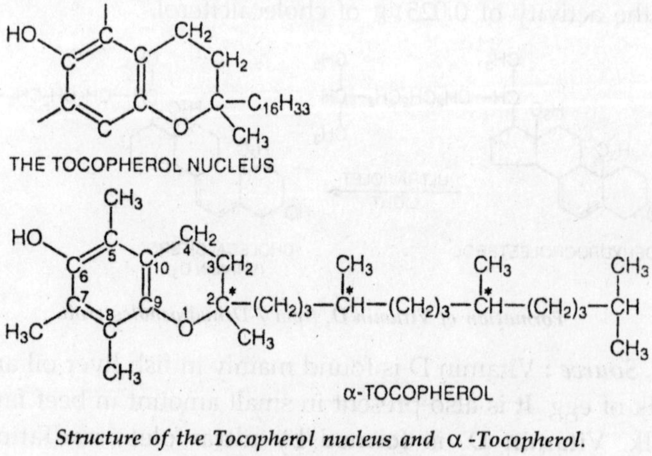

Structure of the Tocopherol nucleus and α-Tocopherol.

Asterisk (*) indicates point of asymmetry.

Source : This vitamin occurs in many foodstuffs, particularly wheat germ. The oils of vegetable seeds (soyabean, cotton, safflower, etc.,) are the richest natural sources of tocopherols. Milk, butter, cheese and meat also have variable and relatively low amount of tocopherol.

Function : The lack of vitamin E causes sterility and death of the embryos in some animals and in rats deficiency produces muscular dystrophy with progressive paralysis of hind legs. Vitamin E plays an essential role in cardiovascular pathology in lower animals. This finding has resulted in attempts to use tocopherols in human therapy.

Some investigators report that cases of angina pectoris, coronary insufficiency, and peripheral vascular diseases improve under tocopherol therapy.

However, the exact physiological role of vitamin E in man is still uncertain, but it may be involved as an anti-oxidant for the preservation of the liquid configuration of cell membranes. All known cases of vitamin E deficiency in human beings are apparently due to defective lipid absorption and transport. In adults, the amount of stored vitamin E is quite high and therefore deficiency may not occur for months or years.

Vitamin K : In 1929-30, *Dam* observed a haemorrhagic syndrome in chicks raised on a diet low in lipids which failed to respond to rich sources of the then known vitamins. In 1935, *Dam* postulated that this syndrome was due to the deficiency of a new fat-soluble vitamin which he called vitamin K (for *Koagulations).*

Vitamin K was isolated in 1939 from alfalfa concentrates and fish meal. The material in alfalfa was designated Vitamin K_1 and that from fish meal K_2. A number of vitamin K_2 analogs are known that differ only in length of the side chain, K_2 from fish meal has 30 carbon atoms.

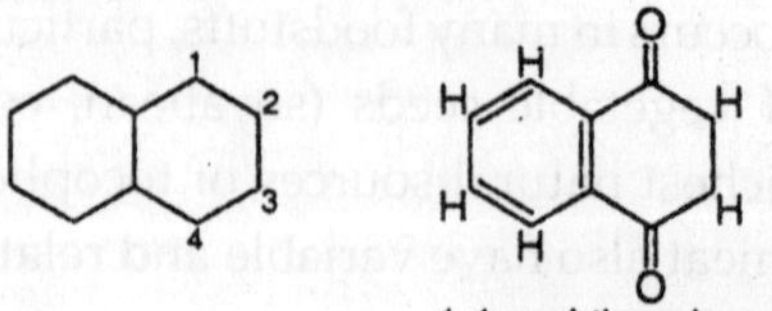

1:4 naphthoquinone

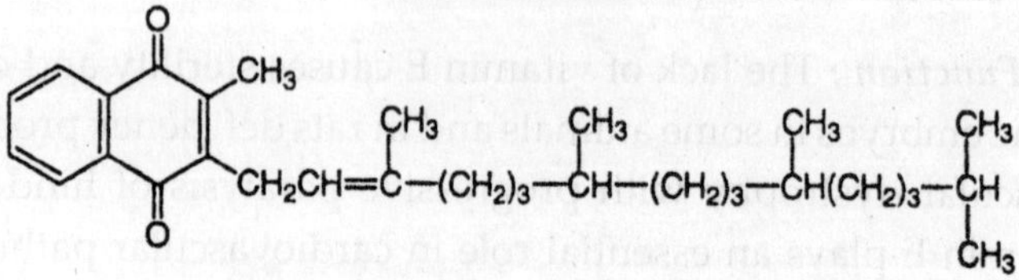

Vitamin K_1 (2-methyl-3-phytyl-1, 4-naphthoquinone)

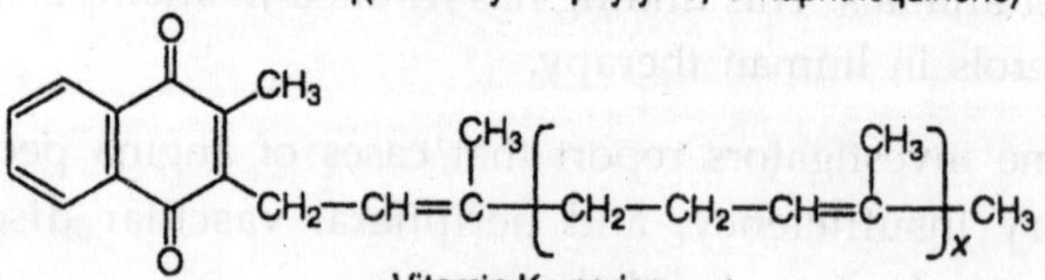

Vitamin K_2 series

Structure of Vitamin K_1 and K_2.

Source : The principal natural sources of vitamin K are green vegetables. This form of the vitamin (K_1) was formerly known as *phylloquinone.*

The vitamin is also present in high concentration in spinach and alfalfa. Soyabean oil, tomatoes, orange peel and hemp seed are also good sources of vitamin K. The bacteria of the human intestine can synthesize vitamin K and probably provide an adequate supply of this vitamin in man.

There are at least two fractions present in natural vitamin K, of which K_1 (Fig.) is more active. It is insoluble in water. However, the synthetic form *menadione* (2-methyl-1, 4-naphthoquinone) is slightly soluble in water.

Function : The absorption of vitamin K from the small intestine takes place only in the presence of adequate amount of bile salts. In the liver it participates in the processes leading to the synthesis of prothrombin and factor VII, IX and X.

Deficiency of vitamin K leads to several clinical conditions including obstructive jaundice, chronic diarrhoea, liver disease, and haemorrhagic disease of the newborn, etc. In the absence of this vitamin the blood clotting time is prolonged and serious haemorrhages may result.

Water-Soluble Vitamins

This class of vitamins includes vitamin B-complex and vitamin C or ascorbic acid.

Vitamin B-Complex : This group consists of a number of water-soluble vitamins, each with a characteristic biological role and a different chemical structure.

They are collectively called the B vitamins because they are often found together in the same food sources, such as liver, yeast, unpolished rice, milk, egg yolk, and green vegetables. The important vitamins of this group are as follows :

(i) Thiamine (B_1)

(ii) Riboflavin (B_2)

(iii) Niacin (Nicotinic acid)

(iv) Pyridoxine (B_6)

(v) Pantothenic acid

(vi) Folic acid

(vii) Biotin

(viii) Cobalamin (Vitamin B_{12})

(ix) Others (Thioctic acid, Para-aminobenzoic acid, Choline, Inositol)

Thiamine

Thiamine (Fig.) is also known as vitamin B_1, Aneurin, Antineuritic factor, Anti-beriberi factor and Oryzanin.

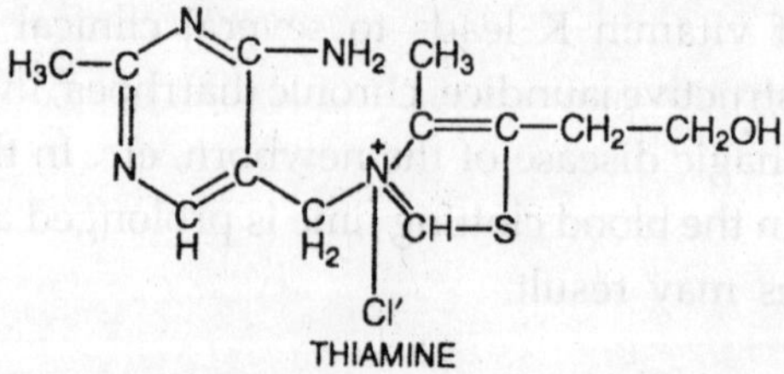

Structure of thiamine consisting of a pyrimidine and a thiazole ring. The molecule is shown as the hydrochloride.

Source : Thiamine is essentially of plant origin and is widely distributed in the seeds, leaves, roots, stems and fruits. In the cereals, thiamine is found mainly in the germ and bran. Leaves and grasses are rich sources of thiamine as are also the beans, nuts, fruits, milk, and egg yolk. However, the presence of thiamine in such products as milk, eggs, and liver depends on the dietary supply of the animal. Of the various meats used by man, pork muscle is the richest in thiamine.

Thiamine occurs in natural products as free thiamine, as a protein complex, as thiamine pyrophosphate (cocarboxylase), and as a phosphorus-protein complex. In milk, it is present both as free thiamine and as the vitamin-protein complex. The approximate daily requirement of vitamin B_1 is 1.5 mg. Normal individuals ingesting 0.5 to 1.5 mg of thiamine daily excrete 50 to 250 μg of this vitamin in the urine. After administration of thiamine to animals, a part may be recovered in the urine unchanged and a part as pyramin.

Function : The main clinical syndrome of thiamine deficiency is known as *beriberi.* The latter has two forms, neuritic or "dry" form in which the spinal cord and peripheral nerves are involved, and cardiac or "wet" form in which the heart is enlarged due to an increase in the weight of the right ventricle. Thiamine lack affecting the brain causes another syndrome known as cerebral beriberi. In all these cases, administration of thiamine in the early stages produces rapid and complete recovery. A characteristic sign of thiamine deficiency in birds is head retraction (opisthotonos), which responds to administration of small quantities of thiamine.

Carbohydrate metabolism in all tissues of the body depends on the presence of a coenzyme thiamine pyrophosphate, which is essential for the decarboxylation of keto acids. Thus, thiamine plays a key role in carbohydrate metabolism. In advanced thiamine deficiency both pyruvic and lactic acids accumulate in the blood whereas glycogen increases in the liver and heart muscle. Diphosphothiamine may be involved in the synthesis of acetylcholine and in the control of its hydrolysis *in vivo*. Thiamine pyrophosphate inhibits the activity of choline esterase of serum.

Riboflavin

Riboflavin is also known as vitamin B_2 or vitamin G. The naturally occurring flavins—lactoflavin, ovoflavin, hepatoflavin, and verdoflavin isolated respectively from milk, egg, liver, and grass, are all chemically identical with riboflavin.

Source : Main dietary sources of riboflavin are liver, kidney, muscle, egg, milk, green leafy vegetables, wheat germ and yeast. It is widely distributed in plant and animal tissues as free riboflavin, as the phosphate, or as the adenine-dinucleotide phosphate. The latter consist of about 70 to 90 per cent of the total riboflavin in tissues. Riboflavin nucleotides occur more or less firmly bound to proteins. The free vitamin is found, for example, in milk, urine and retina. The approximate daily requirement of vitamin B_2 is 1.8 mg. In human beings, excess ingested riboflavin is largely excreted unchanged or as its phosphoric ester (riboflavin -5'-phosphate).

Function : Clinical tests of the riboflavin content of blood and urine have been employed for the diagnosis of riboflavin deficiency. The latter affects primarily the ectodermal tissues, producing lesions of the skin, eye and nervous system. The concentration of riboflavin in erythrocytes is perhaps the most sensitive indicator of its deficiency. Normal whole blood contains 20 μg/dl.

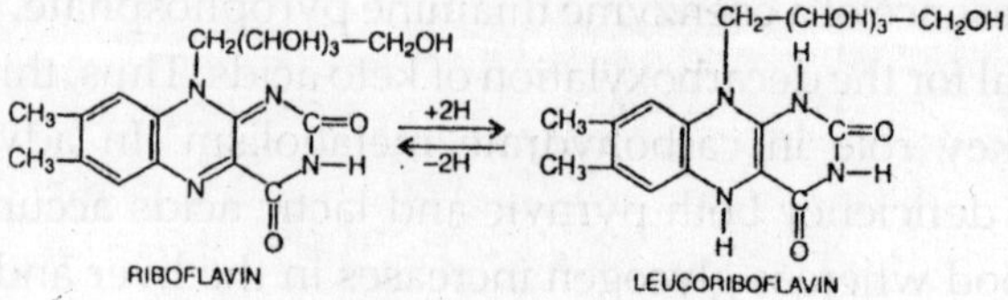

Riboflavin and Leucoriboflavin.

It is well known that the coenzyme derivatives of riboflavin (FMN and FAD) in combination with proteins, are involved in a number of oxidation-reduction reactions. The reduced form of riboflavin is known as leucoriboflavin (Fig.).

It plays a key role in oxidation of hydrogen to water and one would expect that dietary deficiency of riboflavin would lead to serious disturbances in metabolism.

Niacin

Niacin (Fig.) is also known as nicotinic acid, antipellagra factor, and anti-black-tongue factor.

The structure of Niacin (nicotinic acid and nicotinic acid amide).

Source : The richest sources of niacin are liver, fish and meats. The other important sources are wholemeal flour, green vegetables, and cow's milk. The vitamin occurs in relatively high concentration as coenzyme I (NAD) in yeast, red blood cells and heart muscle. The approximate daily requirement of Niacin is 20 μg.

Function : In niacin deficiency, the demonstrable tissue lesions are preceded by functional disturbances which are characteristic of deficiencies of a number of B vitamins. These include weakness, anorexia, indigestion, diarrhoea and mental and emotional disturbances. Following the discovery in 1937 of the importance of niacinamide (nicotinamide) in the nutrition of certain unicellular organisms, the therapeutic effects of nicotinic acid in the treatment of blacktongue and of niacinamide in pellagra were demonstrated.

Niacin was recognised as a component of the coenzymes NADP and NAD in 1935 and 1936 respectively. NAD and NADP are indispensable for many of the energy producing reactions in metabolism. Thus, the metabolic role of Niacin was known before its nutritional significance had been established.

Pyridoxine

Pyridoxine is also known as vitamin B_6, anti-acrodynia factor, and adermin. *Pyridoxol* (Pyridoxine) was isolated from liver and yeast in 1938 and synthesized in the same year. Two other forms of this vitamin, *pyridoxal* and *pyridoxamine* are present in natural sources and the three substances as a group are designated as vitamin B_6 (Fig.).

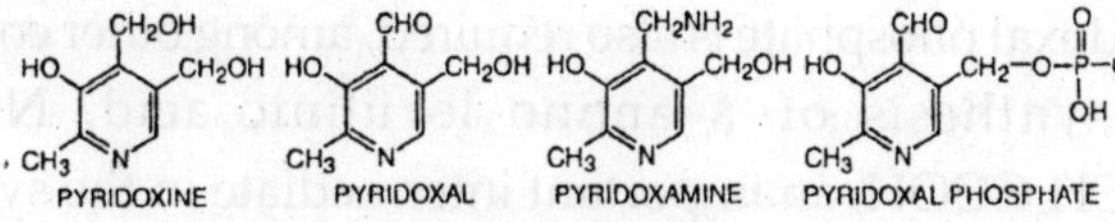

Three components of vitamin B_6 and the coenzyme form pyridoxal phosphate.

Source : Pyridoxol is made in green plants and many microorganisms from 3-carbon derivatives of glycolysis, *e.g.*, glyceraldehyde-3-phosphate. In natural sources, vitamin B_6 is principally bound to proteins. Yeast, rice polishings, the germ of various grains and seeds, and egg yolk are rich sources of this vitamin. Approximate daily requirement of vitamin B_6 is 2 mg. About 90% of the B_6 administered to human is oxidized to 4-pyridoxic acid and excreted in this form.

Function : In rats, deficiency of vitamin B_6 causes acrodynia, edema, growth retardation, nerve degeneration, and abnormal reproductive performance. This vitamin is also essential for the growth of microorganisms, chick, dog, pig, mice and infants.

Vitamin B_6 plays a key role in metabolism. Pyridoxine is essential in the metabolism of fatty acids and in the conversion of protein to fat. Pyridoxal is important in the transport of amino acids and metal ions across the cell membranes. Pyridoxal phosphate is the active form of pyridoxine and acts as the coenzyme in the decarboxylation of several amino acids. The general reaction is :

$$RCHNH_2COOH \longrightarrow RCH_2NH_2 + CO_2$$

Pyridoxal phosphate is also involved as a coenzyme in transaminase reactions and also in the conversion of cysteine to NH_3, H_2S and pyruvic acid, as shown below :

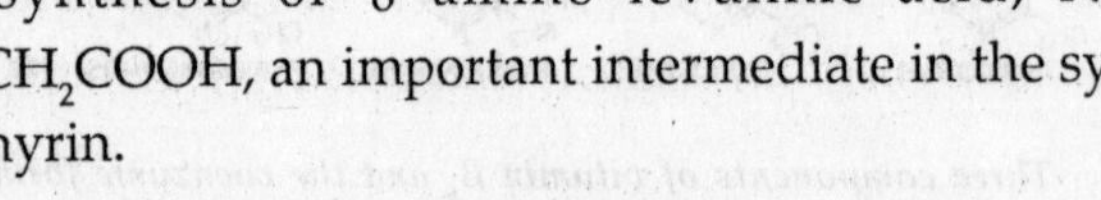

Pyridoxal phosphate is also required, among other cofactors, in the synthesis of δ-amino levulinic acid, $NH_2CH_2COCH_2CH_2COOH$, an important intermediate in the synthesis of porphyrin.

Pantothenic Acid

Pantothenic acid (Fig.) is also known as chick antidermatitis factor and filtrate factor. This factor was first recognized as a portion of the "bios" complex of yeast. Its significance in animal nutrition was established later.

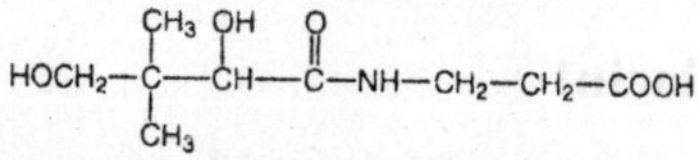

Pantothenic acid.

Source : Pantothenic acid is present in all the living tissues. Liver, kidney, rice bran, egg yolk, peanut and peas are excellent sources of this vitamin. It occurs in natural materials both free and combined, though a major fraction of the vitamin in animal sources is bound. A daily intake of about 5 to 10 mg is probably adequate.

Function : The wide distribution of pantothenic acid in animal and plant tissues is indicative of its fundamental role in metabolism. It is a molecular component of coenzyme A. The latter is the only known functional form of pantothenic acid in microorganisms as well as in animal and plant tissues. Coenzyme A participates in a wide variety of reactions involved in carbohydrate metabolism and fatty acid metabolism. Its acetyl derivative or acetyl CoA has been described by *Welch* and *Nichol* (1952) as the "pivot on which acetyl transfer mechanisms turn". More than 70 enzymes are now known which utilize coenzyme A and acyl carrier protein derivatives.

It is required by chick, rat, pig, dog, and other vertebrates and its deficiency symptoms vary in different species. The lack of dietary pantothenic acid in rats results in necrotic lesions of the adrenal cortex. The deficiency causes increased appetite for salt and a low-salt diet promotes the graying of hair which results from pantothenic acid deficiency. According to *Aiyar* and *Sreenivasan* (1961), the lack of this vitamin produces a decrease in coenzyme Q and succinoxidase activity which is restored to normal after pantothenate administration. *Axelrod* and *Hopper* (1960) have reported that pantothenic acid-deficient rats are unable to produce antibodies in a normal fashion. However, little is known about the relationship between pantothenic acid and antibody response in man.

Folic Acid (Folacin)

Principal synonyms of folic acid are pteroylglutamic acid, folacin, and anti-anemia factor. According to *Angier et al* (1946), the molecule of folic acid consists of a *pteridine* group (I) linked through *p-aminobenzoic acid* (II) to L (+) *glutamic acid* (III). The pteridine linked with *p*-aminobenzoic acid (*i.e.,* portions I and II of the molecule) is termed *pteroic acid* (Fig.). The folic acid produced by *E. coli* and that found in most animal tissues contains predominantly 5 glutamic acid residues combined in γ -glutamyl linkage.

Source : Folic acid is a yellow, tasteless substance, only slightly soluble in water, and widely distributed in common foods in which it is present in various forms including polyglutamic acid conjugates. Yeast, liver, cowpeas, and soyabeans are excellent sources of folic acid. Approximate daily requirement of Folic acid is 50 µg, but because of poor absorption the recommended daily allowance is 400 µg and double this amount is recommended in pregnancy.

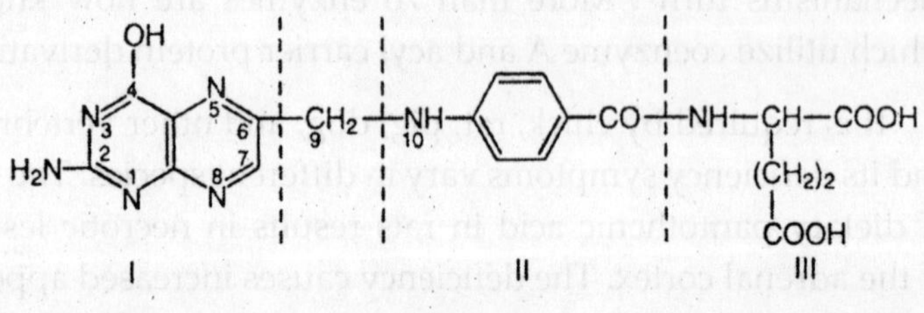

Folic acid

Function : The folic acid as nutritional factor was discovered by the observation that yeast cured a nutritional cytopenia induced in monkeys by corn-containing rations which produce blacktongue in dog. Potent concentrates were obtained from spinach leaf, and this led to the name folic acid (L. *folium*). Folic acid is a growth factor for various microbes, especially the lactic acid bacteria. Its deficiency in animals leads to slow growth and macrocytic anemia. Lack of dietary folic acid in monkeys causes leukopenia, anemia, necrosis of gums, loss of appetite, diarrhoea, and eventual death. Folic acid produces a clinical response in the megaloblastic anemias.

It is used in the treatment of sprue, nutritional megaloblastic anemia and the megaloblastic anemias of pregnancy and infancy. When the hydroxyl in the pteridine ring of folic acid is replaced by an amino group, the resultant *aminopterin* is a folic acid antagonist. Aminopterin and its derivatives are used in the treatment of leukemia, lymphoblastoma and trophoblastic tumors.

One of its derivatives, tetrahydrofolic acid, serves as a carrier of 1-carbon compounds (such as hydroxymethyl and formyl) in much the same fashion as coenzyme A is involved in 2-carbon transfer. It is involved in the synthesis of purines, pyrimidines, and some amino acids. Folic acid is necessary for the normal formation of erythrocytes.

Biotin

Biotin was isolated from egg yolk in 1936. Biotin is also known as vitamin H, anti-egg-white injury factor, Bios II, and coenzyme R.

Source : Biotin occurs in liver, kidney, yeast, cauliflower, peas, and to a lesser extent in many other foodstuffs. It has been isolated as crystalline methyl ester from egg yolk, yeast liver, and milk. Its structure (Fig.) was established by *Vigneaud* as 2-keto-3, 4-imidazolido-2-tetrahydrothiophene-n-valeric acid. In natural products, biotin occurs mainly in bound form. Under ordinary circumstances sufficient quantities of biotin are provided to the mammal by intestinal bacterial synthesis. But the total faecal and urinary excretion of biotin by humans exceeds the dietary intake. On the basis of studies of the biotin requirements of rat, it has been suggested that the daily human metabolic requirement is about 10 μg, but there may be no real requirement for dietary biotin.

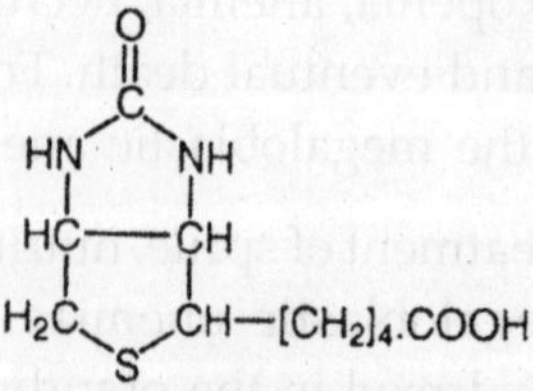

Biotin

Function : Biotin has been shown to be an essential nutrient for various microbes including bacteria, yeast, fungi, and moulds and higher animals (chicken, rat, monkey, man, etc.). Its deficiency in animals is associated with the development of dermatitis, loss of fur, disturbances of the nervous system, and death. Biotin appears to be necessary for normal lactation and gestation in the rat as well as for normal development of chick embryo.

Biotin as prosthetic group of various enzymes plays an important role in metabolism, especially as a key component in carboxylation and decarboxylation reactions involving CO_2, fatty acids, and various dicarboxylic acids. Thus, it participates in such reactions as the interconversion of pyruvic and oxaloacetic acids, of succinic and propionic acids, and of oxalosuccinic and α-ketoglutaric acid; in the synthesis of citrulline from ornithine, of serine from CO_2, and of fatty acids from acetyl coenzyme A. As a coenzyme, biotin is necessary for the fixation of CO_2 into organic substances. In mammals, the biotin side chain undergoes the usual β-oxidation, yielding 2 moles of acetyl coenzyme A. Due to the diversity of its biochemical roles it has been suggested that biotin may act to synthesize specific vitamins rather than participating in their reactions.

Cobalamin

Cobalamin is also called vitamin B_{12}. The structure of vitamin B_{12} is unique as it contains cobalt, which is in the centre of a ring structure. Cyanocobalamin is the form in which vitamin B_{12} is ordinarily available, but the cyanide ion may be replaced by other anions, *e.g.*, hydroxyl, nitrite, chloride, and sulphate. The derivatives are equally active.

The natural vitamins (analogs) are hydroxycobalamin (B_{12} a) and aquocobalamin (B_{12} a, b, d), and synthetic vitamer is nitritocobalamin.

Source : Vitamin B_{12} is absent in plants but present in all animal tissues. It occurs in abundance in liver, kidneys, pancreas, pituitary, and fish. Many microbes including mould of the *streptomyces* group are capable of synthesizing vitamin B_{12}. Ruminants obtain it from fermentations by microflora in the alimentary canal. This accounts for the presence of cobalamins in beef liver and also for the fact that in ruminating animals cobalt deficiency leads to a wasting disease caused by a lack of vitamin B_{12}. Approximate daily requirement of cobalamin is 1 to 3 μg.

Function : It is essential for normal growth and reproduction in a number of laboratory animals. It is essential for the maintenance of good health in humans. It is necessary for development of erythrocytes, especially for the maturation of nucleated red cells (erythroblasts). Deficiency of vitamin B_{12} in humans causes *pernicious anaemia*. This megaloblastic anaemia is usually associated with severe involvement of the central nervous system and the gastro-intestinal mucosa. This disease is due to lack of *'intrinsic factor'* (or gastric factor, which is present in gastric juice) with a consequent failure in the absorption of vitamin B_{12}.

Vitamin C (Ascorbic Acid) : Vitamin C is also a water-soluble vitamin. *Szent-Gyorgyi* (1928, 1932) named vitamin C as "ascorbic acid" because of its antiscorbutic properties. It was first isolated in crystalline form from lemon juice by *King* and *Waugh* (1932).

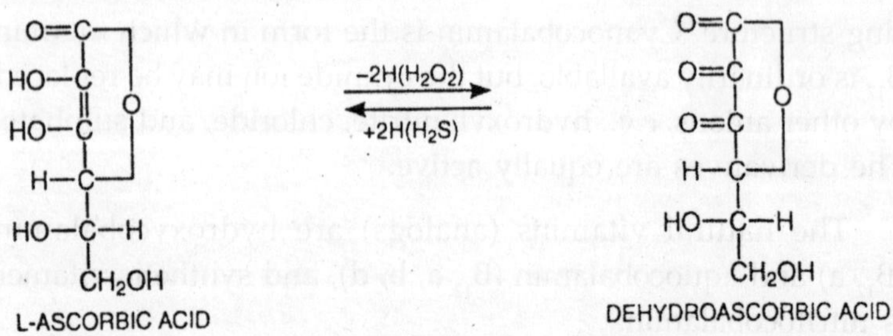

Ascorbic acid

Source : Fresh fruits and vegetables are excellent sources of vitamin C. Special mention may be made of cabbage, cauliflower, kohlrobi spinach, parsley, kale, broccoli, cresses, peppers, oranges, lemons, grapefruit, tangerines, limes, strawberries, and gooseberries. Vitamin C content of human milk is considerably higher than that of cow's milk.

Vitamin C is a strong reducing agent (Fig.) and therefore readily oxidised. In an alkaline medium destruction by oxygen is rapid at 100°C. It is therefore generally absent from dried, canned, or preserved foods unless they are processed anaerobically. During the cooking of vegetables, vitamin C is lost by over-cooking.

Function : Vitamin C acts as a cofactor for the hydroxylation of certain proteins. The only species that depend on dietary sources for vitamin C are humans, guinea-pigs, and monkeys. Many other animals contain vitamin C in their tissues but synthesize it for themselves.

Deficiency of vitamin C in susceptible species causes a painful disease of joints and gums called *Scurvy*. Scurvy in adults is characterized by sore, spongy gums, loosening of the teeth, impaired capillary integrity with subcutaneous haemorrhages and edema, joint pain, anorexia, and anaemia. In severe scurvy there is failure of formation of new ground substance and extensive depolymerization and solution of existing cement material, leading to breakdown of old, healed wounds. The biochemical lesions which cause scurvy are unknown, as is the precise role of vitamin C in metabolism, though it is probably concerned with the maintenance of connective tissue in general and intercellular ground substance, capillary lining and bone matrix in particular.

The useful effects of vitamin C in developing body resistance to cold and tissue-healing are well known. Recently it has been shown that vitamin C has virucidal activity (virus killing) and its effectiveness in the therapy of measles and mumps is also receiving attention of scientists. *Banic* (1975) has also reported the preventive effect of vitamin C in rabies infection in guinea pigs. Approximate daily requirement of ascorbic acid

Names, Sources and Effects of Deficiency of Vitamins

S.No.	Name	Main sources	Chief cellular functions	Effects of deficiency
1.	Vitamin A	Carotenes, liver oils	Plays a role in the chemistry of vision	Night blindness, infectious diseases, bone and nerve abnormalities.
2.	Vitamin D	Milk, egg yolk, liver, fish oils	Regulation of Calcium & Phosphorous	Rickets.
3.	Vitamin E	Green leafy vegetables, oils from seeds, egg yolk, meat	H transfer during aerobic respiration	Sterility, eye abnormalities, nerve and muscle disorders
4.	Vitamin K	Green leafy vegetables, egg yolk liver	H transfer during aerobic respiration, synthesis of prothrombin in liver.	Failure of blood clotting,
5.	Vitamin B Complex			
(i)	Thiamine (B_1)	Egg, meat, liver, beans, yeast, cereals	Precursor of cocarboxylase (thiamine pyrophosphate)	Beriberi, Polyneuritis (inflammation and degeneration of nerves).
(ii)	Riboflavin (B_2)	Vegetables, yeast, milk, liver, egg	Precursor of FMN and FAD	Loss of hair, inflammation of eyes
(iii)	Niacin or Nicotinic acid	Yeast, meat, egg	Precursor of NAD and NADP	Pellagra (a disease affecting skin, alimentary canal and nerves)
(iv)	Pantothenic acid	Yeast, meat, egg, grain	Precursor of coenzyme A	
(v)	Folic acid	—do—	Nucleic acid metabolism	Anaemia, growth failure, haemorrhages, disorders of bone and skin, infectious diseases.
(vi)	Cobalamin (B_{12})	—do—	—do—	
(vii)	Biotin (H)	—do—	—do—	—do—
(viii)	Choline	—do—	—do—	
(ix)	Pyridoxine (B_6)	—do—	—do—	
6.	Vitamin C	Citrus fruits, tomatoes, cabbage	H transfer during aerobic respiration, synthesis of cell cement	Scurvy.

is 45 μg . The normal human plasma ascorbic acid concentration is 0.7 to 1.2 μg /dl. Evaluation of ascorbic acid deficiency is sometimes made by estimates of the level in platelets. Scurvy

is usually evident when the ascorbic acid level is less than 25% of the normal value of 52 ± 22 μg per 10^{10} platelets.

The names, food-sources, functions and the clinical effects of the deficiency of vitamins are summarized in Table.

Choline

It is sometimes included in the water-soluble vitamins. Choline and inositol are sometimes classed as B vitamins. This is because neither is synthesized to a sufficient extent by animal cells. It is constituent of *lecithin* (one of cell phospholipids). A deficiency of choline produces symptoms (hemorrhaging of kidneys and deposition of excess fat in the liver) similar to those induced by a lack of amino acid, *methionine*. Thus, choline and methionine serve as the source of certain simple chemical groupings called methyl (CH_3–) groups in cell metabolism.

$$\begin{array}{l} CH_2CH_2OH \\ | \\ N(CH_3)_3 \end{array}$$

Choline

Presumably, the demand for choline and methionine is influenced by the amount of folic acid and vitamin B_{12} present in the diet. Choline is widely distributed as a constituent of phosphatidyl choline and glandular tissues are excellent dietary sources as are nervous tissue, egg, yolk, and a few vegetable oils, *e.g.*, soyabean oil.

Purines and Pyrimidines

These bases are essential for the biosynthesis of nucleic acids (DNA and RNA).

Sterols : Steroids are a large class of fused carbon ring compounds. The most common of animal sterols is *cholesterol*. This is important in the synthesis of fatty acids and of some steroid hormones. Apparently, all animals use cholesterol in lipid metabolism, but there are variations in their ability to synthesize it.

Feeding Mechanisms of Animals **:** The intake of food is called *feeding*. The method of feeding appears to be determined largely by the habitat and the food available to a particular organism. In most cases the form and function of the digestive tract also depends upon the types of food and feeding mechanism. According to *CM. Yonge* (1928), the feeding mechanisms of animals belong to the following three categories *(a, b, c)*.

(a) Mechanisms for Dealing with Small Particles

Minute particles in the form of detritus, diatoms, flagellates, and bacteria, are used as food by a large number of sessile or sluggish aquatic animals. They collect the food particles by any of the following methods :

1. *Pseudopodial Feeding* : Feeding by the use of pseudopodia is a characteristic of the rhizopods. In *Amoeba,* the food is captured by the pseudopodia which extend around the food particle and engulf it together with some amount of water. Particles are caught by the reticulate pseudopodia of radiolarians and foraminiferans and then brought to the main part of the body for digestion.

2. *Mucoid Feeding* : Many animals secrete mucous sheets which filter out particles, which are then eaten by the animals. The tube-living polychaete, *Chaetopterus* and the echiuroid worm, *Urechis,* secrete a mucous net, pump water through it by the activity of posterior appendages and swallow the trapped food. An interesting example of mucoid feeding is provided by a sessile gastropod, *Vermetus.* Some protochordates also have a mucous-ciliary type of feeding, in which food particles entangled in mucous are ingested by the animal.

3. *Ciliary and Flagellar Feeding* : This mechanism is commonly used by a large number of sedentary animals like the ciliate protozoans, sponges, many tubiculous annelids, lamellibranchs, and many tunicates and cephalochordates. In most of such animals the beating of cilia or flagella continuously produces the respiratory cum feeding currents of water and helps in directing the food particles towards the mouth.
4. *Tentacular and Setose Feeding* : Some animals depend largely upon their freely movable ciliated tentacles for collecting food particles. In certain coelenterates the nematocysts on the tentacles help to paralyse the prey which is often attached to the tentacles by a sticky secretion. In some crustaceans, the setae (hair like chitinous structures) on various appendages are used to create the currents of water. Copepods produce currents by antennal vibrations.

(b) Mechanisms for Dealing with Large Particles (or masses)

Some burrowing animals swallow *inactive food* such as mud. Certain holothurians use their tentacles to force mud into their digestive tracts. Annelids such as *Lumbricus* and *Arenicola* use their reversible pharynx for this purpose. The organic content of the mud is utilized and the residue ejected as faeces.

Some animals have structures *for scraping and boring* food stuffs. Examples are the Aristotle's lantern of echinoid echinoderms, radular apparatus of some molluscs, boring valves of the shipworm *Teredo,* and heavy mouth parts of termites.

In certain animals specialized organs serve to seize the prey. They may be for seizing only as the protruded proboscis of *Didinium,* the jawed pharynx of many polychaetes, and the teeth of a shark, etc. The other category of such organs are the *structures for seizing and masticating.* Examples are the jaws and radulas of molluscs, the jaws and other mouth parts of crustaceans, insects, arachnids and myriapods, and the toothed jaws of vertebrates. In the jawed vertebrates the anterior teeth often bite or gnaw, posterior teeth masticate. However, there is much variation ranging from amphibians and billed birds which chew very little to the ungulates with heavy chewing molars.

A third category of the prey-feeding mechanism employs the *structures for seizing followed by external digestion.* An interesting example of this is furnished by the sacrodinian, *Vampyrella,* which digests a hole through the walls of the algae on which its feeds. Some carnivorous gastropods, cephalopods, spiders and echinoderms seize their prey and also carry out some external digestion.

(c) Mechanisms for Taking in Fluids (liquid food)

Some parasitic animals feed on fluids and soft tissues. The structures for *piercing* and *sucking* are found in hookworms, leeches, ticks, mites and cyclostomes. The structures for *sucking* only are met with in suctorian protozoans, nematodes, adult butterflies and suckling mammals. The endoparasites such as sporozoans, cestodes and *Sacculina,* depend on the absorption of the nutrient materials from the internal body surface of their hosts.

Regulation of Food Intake

Humans regulate their food intake by an interesting feedback mechanism. Now it is known that the hypothalamus influences the food intake and the body weight. The *ventrolateral* and the *ventromedial* nuclei in the hypothalamus are considered as being facilitatory and inhibitory centres. The inhibitory centre, also called the *satiety centre,* is said to function by inhibiting the lateral nuclei. The lateral nuclei, referred to as the *feeding centre* (hunger centre), in some way gives rise to hunger. Thus, the *hypothalamic theory of food intake* states that we eat in response to the activity of the hunger centre. When one has eaten adequately the satiety centre becomes active and thereby inhibits the hunger centre, and eating stops.

Experiments have shown that the *blood glucose* is the critical factor that stimulates one or the other of the two centres. If the blood reaching the brain contains a high glucose level, the satiety centre probably responds selectively to this level and issues the command "do not eat". Conversely, low glucose levels probably stimulate the hunger centre selectively and result in the command "eat". Thus, any condition or factor that directly or indirectly influences the glucose delivery to the brain, or affects the hypothalamus, is bound to affect the food intake.

3

Digestion System

Digestion can be defined as a *process that involves chemical breakdown of complex food materials into simpler molecules which can be readily used by the animal through absorption and assimilation.*

Kinds of Digestion

Intracellular Digestion : When digestion takes place inside the cells and is carried out in food vacuoles within the organism itself, then it is called intracellular digestion. This mode of digestion is a characteristic of lower animals like protozoans and sponges. However, it is also employed by some more complex animals like coelenterates wherein the digestion is partially extracellular but largely intracellular. Many platyhelminths and *Limulus* are also considered as examples of animals in which the occurrence of intracellular digestion represents a primitive condition.

Extracellular Digestion : When digestion is practically completed in the lumen of the digestive tract, it is called extracellular digestion. Thus, the development of a digestive tract, permits a more complete extracellular digestion, which is a characteristic of higher animals like crustaceans, insects, cephalopods, tunicates and all vertebrates.

Mechanical Factors in Digestion : The digestive tracts of animals show striking adaptations to the kind of food and the feeding habits of the organism. The digestive tract usually consists of the following functional regions : (a) the region of reception of food, (b) the region of conduction and storage, (c) the region of internal trituration and early digestion, (d) the region of final digestion and absorption and (e) the region of faeces formation.

Movement of Food Mass

The food is propelled along the digestive tract by ciliary action, or by muscular activity, or by a combination of both. The ciliary action takes place in such organisms as the ectoprocts, endoprocts and pelecypod molluscs. The muscular activity or the so-called *peristalsis* is found in other animals, including vertebrates. In addition to moving the food, the muscular activity also serves to triturate the food and to mix the food with digestive fluids.

Thus, the main functions of the digestive system may be described as follows:

1. Ingestion of food
2. Digestion of food
3. Secretion of digestive juices and enzymes
4. Movements of the gastro-intestinal tract facilitate mixing of food with digestive juices; propel food onwards, and are responsible for defaecation.
5. The alimentary canal takes part in the regulation of blood reaction through alternate acid and alkaline reaction of digestive juices, and also in the regulation of blood sugar.

6. Absorption of water, salts, vitamins, and end products of food digestion.
7. Maintenance of water balance of the body through the phenomenon of thirst.

Digestive Enzymes

Digestive enzymes play an important role in digestion as they regulate (mediate) the chemical reactions in the breakdown of food. Most digestive enzymes are *Hydrolases* and produce their catalytic action by the process of *Hydrolysis* (Fig.), in which a molecule of

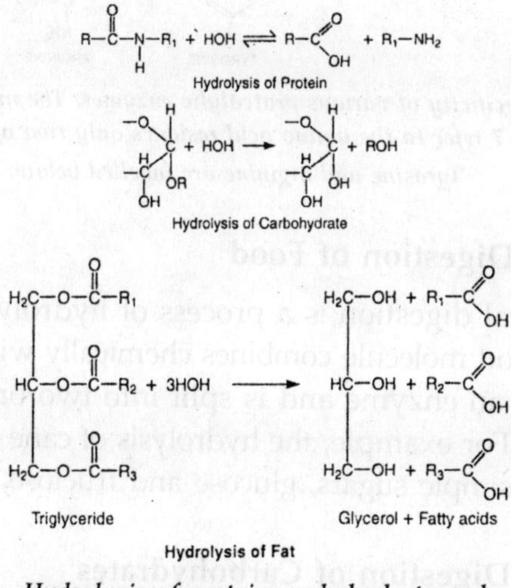

Hydrolysis of protein, carbohydrate and fat by the addition of the elementss of water. The R represents a complex carbon skeleton.

water is chemically added to the food molecule, which then separates (splits) into two or more smaller molecules. In hydrolysis, cleavage may involve several stages before the final molecules are obtained. In proteins, for example, the first stage in hydrolysis will yield proteoses (molecules of several amino acids), and additional hydrolytic reactions will be necessary before amino acids will be split off. Before they can be absorbed, proteins must be split into amino acids, carbohydrates into more simple sugars, and fats into glycerol and fatty acids. Specific enzymes for each of these processes are found in various regions of the alimentary canal. One enzyme may finish what another (the predecessor) has started.

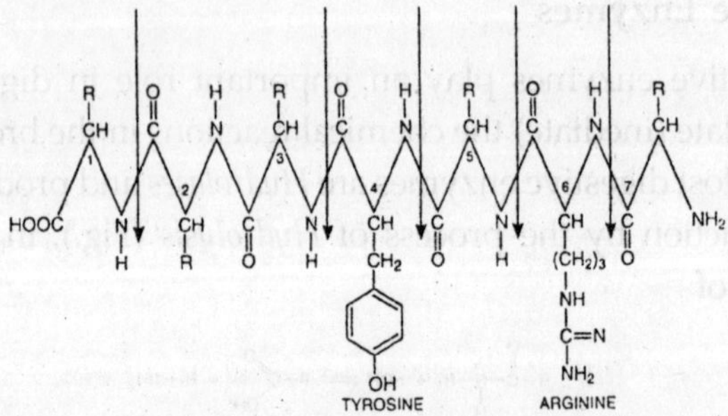

Specificity of various proteolylic enzymes. The numbers 1 to 7 refer to the amino acid residues only two of which, tyrosine and arginine are labelled below.

Chemical Digestion of Food

Chemical digestion is a process of hydrolysis in which a complex food molecule combines chemically with water in the presence of an enzyme and is split into two or more simpler molecules. For example, the hydrolysis of cane sugar (sucrose) yields two simple sugars, glucose and fructose.

Chemical Digestion of Carbohydrates

Simple sugars (monosaccharides) are soluble in water. They can be absorbed in the intestine without further change, and consequently are not digested. Disaccharides and polysaccharides are hydrolyzed during digestion into two simple sugars and many simple sugars respectively. One molecule of a disaccharide when hydrolyzed with one molecule of water in the presence of an appropriate enzyme, gives two monosaccharides as follows:

$$\underset{\text{Disaccharide (Sucrose)}}{C_{12}H_{22}O_{11}} + H_2O \xrightarrow{\textit{sucrase}} \underset{\text{Glucose}}{C_6H_{12}O_6} + \underset{\text{Fructose}}{C_6H_{12}O_6}$$

When polysaccharides are hydrolyzed, they break up into many simple sugars. For example, the hydrolysis of *starch* yields several molecules of *dextrin,* which is then hydrolyzed into the disaccharide maltose, and this into the monosaccharide glucose.

The chemical digestion or hydrolysis of carbohydrates occurs in the presence of different enzymes known as *glycosidases.* Two enzymes, ptyalin and maltase are present in the saliva. *Ptyalin* or salivary amylase hydrolyzes starch to dextrin and maltose, and then *maltase* converts maltose to glucose. Enzymes secreted by the small intestine continue the process : *maltase* hydrolyzes maltose to glucose, *invertase* (sucrase) acts upon sucrose and hydrolyzes it to glucose and fructose, and *lactase* hydrolyzes lactose (milk sugar) to glucose and galactose. Glucose, fructose, and galactose are all simple sugars that can be absorbed into the blood.

Chemical Digestion of Proteins

In addition to the dietary proteins, about 10 to 30 g of protein are present in various digestive juices and another 10 g of protein are contained in cells desquamated each day from the intestinal lining. This protein is also digested and absorbed. The digestion of the protein by a proteolytic enzyme occurs by the hydrolysis of peptide bonds and the protein is digested according to the following sequence :

$$\text{Protein} \rightarrow \text{proteoses} \rightarrow \text{peptones} \rightarrow \text{polypeptides} \rightarrow \text{amino acids}$$

No protein digestion occurs in the mouth. In the stomach *pepsin* hydrolyzes proteins into proteoses and peptones. In the small intestine the enzyme *trypsin* from the pancreas converts proteins and partially digested proteins into polypeptides. Finally, in the small intestine the enzyme *erepsin* further acts upon the split products of the gastric digestion of proteins to form amino acids which can be absorbed.

In the complete hydrolysis of a polypeptide, only carbonyl-to-nitrogen bonds are ruptured (see arrows in the following reaction). A hydroxyl group, from water becomes attached to each carbonyl carbon, and a hydrogen atom (also from water) becomes attached to each nitrogen.

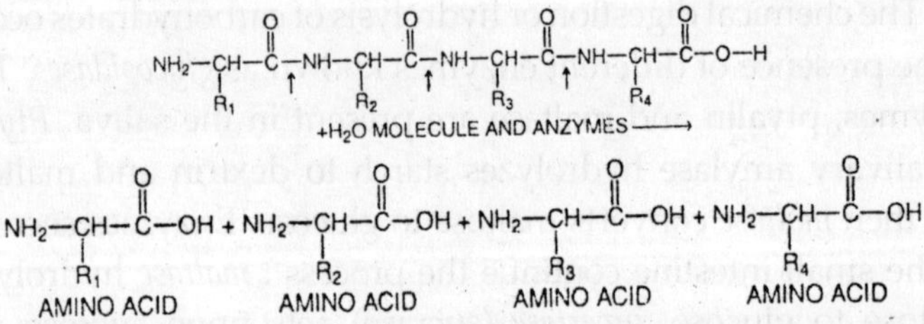

It should be noted that a protein molecule is split first by *endopeptidases* (pepsin, chymotrypsin, and trypsin) into smaller fragments from the ends of which amino acids are hydrolyzed by the *exopeptidases* (aminopolypeptidases, carboxy-polypeptidases). The latter perform their work more effectively after the action of endopeptidases, since more ends of protein fragments then become available for their action.

The high degree of the specificity of various proteolytic enzymes is shown by the fact that each of them attacks a particular linkage between amino acids (Fig.). *Pepsin* attacks a protein (or protein fragment) on the amino side of the peptide bond between tyrosine (or phenylalanine) and other amino acids. *Chymotrypsin* attacks the carboxyl end of the bond between tryosine (or phenylalanine, tryptophan, and methionine) and other amino acids. *Trypsin* acts at the carboxyl end of arginine or lysine residue (*Cantarow* and *Schepartz*, 1967).

Similarly, expopeptidases are also specific in their action. *Aminopolypeptidases* attack a polypeptide on the end where a free amino group exists. *Carboxypolypeptidases* attack a polypeptide on the end where a free carboxyl group is present. The result of each reaction is the production of a free amino acid and a polypeptide molecule with reduced molecular weight. Many *dipeptidases* probably exist, each one specific to a particular dipeptide (*Smith*, 1960).

Chemical Digestion of Fats

Enzymatic hydrolysis of fat converts it into smaller molecules: glycerol and fatty acids. For example, the fat known as *stearin* hydrolyzes as follows:

$$\underset{\text{stearin}}{C_3H_5O_3(C_{17}H_{35}CO)_3} + \underset{\text{water}}{3H_2O} \xrightarrow{\text{lipase}} \underset{\text{1 glycerol}}{C_3H_5(OH)_3} + \underset{\text{3 stearic acid}}{{}_3HC_{18}H_{35}O_2}$$

The digestion of fat starts in the stomach, no digestion of fat occurring in the mouth. The *lipase* of the gastric juice acts on emulsified fats such as cream. Most fat is digested in the small intestine. In the duodenum, the bolus of food encounters the bile and the pancreatic juice. The presence of lipid in the small intestine stimulates the release of the gastro-intestinal hormone cholecystokinin. This decreases gastric motility so that the gastric contents are released more slowly. Cholecystokinin also stimulates lipase secretion by the pancreas and contraction of the gall bladder to release bile into the small intestine. The enzyme lipase from the pancreas (the so-called pancreatic lipase or steapsin) splits fats into glycerol and fatty acids that can be absorbed. However, the bile from the liver breaks up the fat droplets into small ones (emulsification) and thus hastens the action of lipase.

Digestion in Vertebrates

The process of digestion in vertebrates consists of a series of hydrolyses and follows more or less a similar course in all of them. The structural plan of the alimentary canal among the various vertebrates is quite similar and consists of the following essential regions: mouth, buccal cavity, pharynx, oesophagus, stomach, and small and large intestines. In addition, there are several digestive glands. The salivary glands secrete saliva into the mouth cavity. The liver and the exocrine pancreas empty their secretions into the small intestine (duodenum). In a higher vertebrate (particularly humans), the digestion can be discussed under the following heads.

Digestion in the Mouth

In the mouth, the food is broken down mechanically by teeth and chemically by certain enzymes. The food is, thus, masticated and mixed with saliva secreted by the salivary glands. The saliva contains water, mucous, and a digestive enzyme called the salivary amylase *(ptyalin)* that acts on starch. Salivary α -amylase occurs as a mixture of closely related iso-enzymes. Each is a single chain polypeptide (MW = 56,000) to which is attached an oligosaccharide. In humans, the saliva also contains an enzyme, *maltase* in traces. The pH optimum of the salivary amylase is neutral or slightly alkaline. It splits starch and other complex carbohydrates into maltose which is broken down by *maltase* into glucose.

There are no digestive juices secreted into the oesophagus, and the food simply passes through the oesophagus to the stomach.

Digestion in the Stomach

The food is subjected to both muscular movements and chemical reactions in the stomach. The gastric glands in the wall of the stomach secrete *gastric juice* (Fig.). The gastric glands consist of 3 kinds of cells : *chief cells* filled with secretory granules containing pepsinogen, *Oxyntic* (parietal) *cells* which secrete hydrochloric acid, and *mucous* cells which secrete mucous. The fasting stomach of humans secretes about 8 to 15 ml of gastric juice in 24 hr. Gastric and duodenal ulcers result from the digestion of mucosa by pepsin and HCl. Thus, gastric juice is composed of water, mucin, salts, hydrochloric acid and three enzymes, *pepsin, rennin* and fat-splitting *gastric lipase*. The pepsin is secreted in the form of its zymogen precursor *pepsiongen* and rennin in the form of *prorennin*. The hydrochloric acid performs several functions in the stomach. First, it kills several bacteria that are swallowed with the food. It converts pepsinogen into active pepsin and provides an acidic medium for the action of pepsin. The low pH caused by the hydrochloric acid is also responsible for the precipitation of many soluble proteins, so that they can remain in the stomach for a longer time to be broken down by the pepsin.

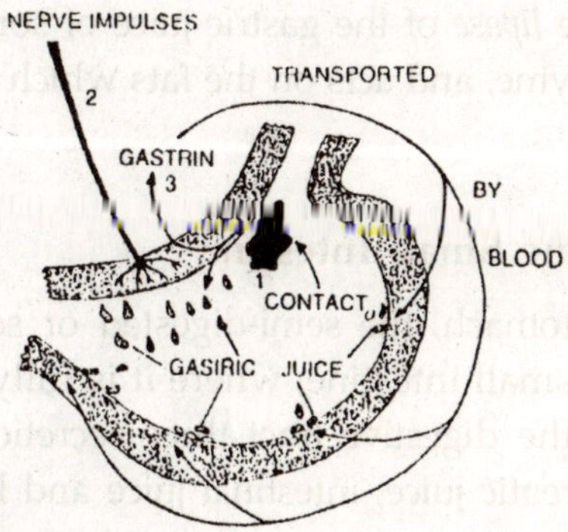

The three processes by which the stomach lining may be stimulated to secrete gastric juice. 1. by contact with food, 2. by nerve impulses from the brain, and 3. by the hormone gastrin.

Pepsin : It is a protein-splitting or proteolytic enzyme. The precursor pepsinogen (MW = 42,500) is converted into pepsin (MW = 35,000) both by the acidity of the gastric juice and by pepsin itself. During this conversion, 42 amino acid residues are removed from the NH_2-terminal end of pepsinogen as a mixture of peptides. The pH optimum of pepsin is about 2 and the enzyme, therefore, works well in the acidic gastric juice. Pepsin digests proteins up to the stage of peptone.

Rennin : It acts by splitting the milk protein *(caseinogen)* into two smaller fragments called *casein* and *whey* (the watery part of milk). The casein combines with the calcium usually found in the milk to form an insoluble calcium protein or *curd*. As a result of this *curding*, the milk proteins are retained in the stomach long enough for pepsin to act on them. The abomasum (fourth stomach) of ruminants contains a protease, *chymosin* (formerly *rennin),* that hydrolyzes *casein* (the principal protein of bovine milk) to *paracasein* which then reacts with Ca^{2+} to yield the insoluble curd. Chymosin is not present in the human stomach. However, pepsin can also catalyze the conversion of casein to paracasein. This is the initial step in casein digestion in the infant stomach.

Lipase : The *lipase* of the gastric juice of some animals is a fat-splitting enzyme, and acts on the fats which are in very fine emulsion.

Digestion in the Small Intestine

From the stomach, the semi-digested or semi-liquid food passes into the small intestine, where it is fully digested. Into this region of the digestive tract three secretions are poured. These are pancreatic juice, intestinal juice and bile.

(i) Pancreatic Juice

It contains sodium carbonate and the following enzymes.

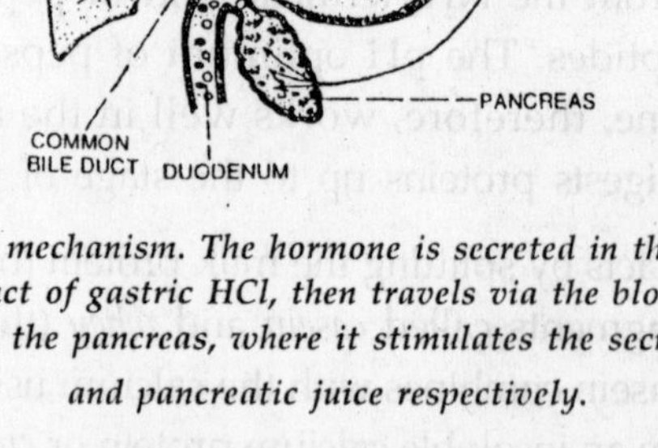

The secretin mechanism. The hormone is secreted in the duodenum by the contact of gastric HCl, then travels via the bloodstream to the liver and the pancreas, where it stimulates the secretion of bile and pancreatic juice respectively.

(a) *Trypsin :* This is secreted in an inactive form called *trypsinogen* and is activated by another enzyme *enteropeptidase* (previously called *enterokinase)* from the intestinal wall. Trypsinogen consists of a single peptide chain and its conversion into trypsin involves scission of a single bond, liberating the NH_2—terminal hexapeptide from the zymogen molecule. Trypsin acts upon natural proteins and splits them to proteoses and peptones.

(b) *Chymotrypsin* : This is also secreted in an inactive form known as *chymotrypsinogen,* and is activated into chymotrypsin by trypsin. Chymotrypsin also acts upon proteins, converting them into peptides, and clots milk.

(c) *Carboxypeptidase* : The protein digestion is further enhanced by carboxypeptidase which acts upon already formed peptides, and splits them into free amino acids. *Carboxypeptidase A*, a zinc-containing enzyme, rapidly liberates COOH-terminal residues possessing aromatic or aliphatic side chains. *Carboxypeptidase B* acts only on peptides with terminal arginine or lysine residues.

(d) *Elastase*: Elastase attacks peptide bonds involving neutral aliphatic amino acids.

(e) *Amylase or Amylopsin:* Pancreatic amylase (α-1,4-glucan-4 glucano hydrolase) is an endoenzyme which hydrolyzes interior α-1, 4 bonds of polysaccharides. Digestion of *amylose* yields *maltose* and *maltotriose.* Pancreatic amylase also hydrolyzes *amylopectin* which represents about 80% starch consumed by human beings. These reactions are summarised as follows:

$$\underset{\text{(α-1, 4-linked glucose units)}}{\text{Amylose}} \xrightarrow{\text{α amylase}} \text{maltotriose} + \text{maltose}$$

$$\underset{\text{(α-1, 4-linked glucose units and α-1, 6-linked units)}}{\text{Amylopectin}} \xrightarrow{\text{α amylase}} \underset{\text{(5-10 glucose residues)}}{\text{α-limit dextrins}}$$

(f) *Pancreatic Lipase or Steapsin* : It is a lipolytic enzyme and converts fats into fatty acids and glycerol. The mechanism of action of pancreatic lipase is unique. The main products of its action on triacyl glycerols are the fatty acids and the 2-monoacyl glycerols and each enzyme molecule can split 4×10^5 ester bonds per minute.

Thus, the substrate for its action is present in lipid phase, whereas the water molecules required for rapid hydrolysis are present in the aqueous phase. The enzymatic reaction occurs at the oil-water interface. Two other components also facilitate this reaction. These are bile salts and a *colipase* secreted into the pancreatic juice. Bile salts help to emulsify fat into particles with an increased total surface area available for lipase action. *Colipase* is a polypeptide which helps to anchor the enzyme in an active form to the surface of the fat droplet, where the hydrolysis occurs.

Bile salts and colipase also shift the optimum pH of pancreatic lipase from 8.5 to 6.0. Since the pH of the upper small intestine is between 6 and 6.5, this increases enzyme activity.

(g) *Other Pancreatic Enzymes* : In addition to the above enzymes, pancreatic juice also contains *maltase* and *ribonuclease*. The former splits maltose into glucose, whereas the latter is responsible for the hydrolysis of RNA to smaller nucleotides. Pancreatic juice also contains *esterases* that can hydrolyze short-chain fatty acid esters, *e.g.*, tributyrin.

These esterases have an absolute requirement for bile salts. There is also a *cholesterol esterase*, which hydrolyzes cholesterol esters to fatty acids and cholesterol. *Prophospholipase* A_2 is produced in the pancreas and is activated by trypsin to produce *phospholipase* A_2, which is active only in the presence of Ca^{2+} and bile salts. The enzyme liberates a fatty acid from the 2 position of phosphatidylcholine to produce lysophosphatidyl choline. The latter aids in emulsification of the dietary lipid.

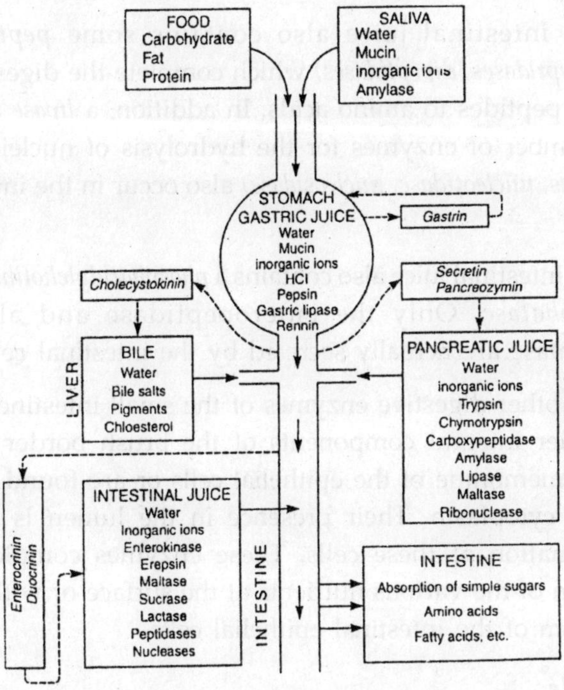

The physiology of mammalian digestion (diagrammatric).

(ii) Intestinal Juice

In addition to the *enterokinase* mentioned above, the *succus entricus* (intestinal secretion) contains several enzymes which are necessary to complete the gastric digestion. One of these, *erepsin,* completes the gastric digestion of peptones and proteoses, and splits them into amino acids.

The other enzymes are concerned with carbohydrate splitting. *Maltase* converts maltose into glucose, *Sucrase* splits sucrose to glucose and fructose, and *lactase* breaks down *lactose* (milk sugar) into glucose and galactose. The acid contents from the stomach also cause the intestinal mucosa to release the hormone, *secretin,* which carried in the blood to the pancreas, stimulates the flow of pancreatic juice.

The intestinal juice also contains some *peptidases, (aminopeptidases, dipeptidases)* which complete the digestion of various peptides to amino acids. In addition, a *lipase* as well as a number of enzymes for the hydrolysis of nucleic acids *(nucleases, nucleotidase, nucleosidase)* also occur in the intestinal juice.

The intestinal juice also contains a *phosphatidylcholinase* and a *phosphatase.* Only the enteropeptidase and alkaline phosphatase are actually secreted by the intestinal cells.

The other digestive enzymes of the small intestine are in fact either integral components of the brush border of the plasma membrane of the epithelial cells or are found within the cell cytoplasm. Their presence in the lumen is due to desquamation of these cells. These enzymes complete the digestion of the various nutrients at the surface or within the cytoplasm of the intestinal epithelial cells.

(iii) Bile

It is made up of water, bile salts and certain pigments. Bile is usually stored in the gall bladder and is stimulated to flow down the common bile duct when food enters the small intestine. A hormone, *cholecystokinin,* secreted by the intestinal lining, plays a part in regulating the flow of bile because it stimulates contraction of the gall bladder. Bile salts emulsify fat into small particles so that the fat-splitting enzymes may have a chance to reduce them. By virtue of its alkaline nature bile creates a suitable medium for intestinal digestion. The *bile salts* are formed in the liver cells in a manner analogous to the formation of hippuric acid :

$$\text{Cholic acid} + \text{CoA} + \text{ATP} \rightarrow \text{Cholyl CoA} + \text{AMP} + \text{PPi}$$

$$\text{Cholyl CoA} + \text{Glycine} \rightarrow \text{Cholylglycine} + \text{CoA}$$

In the bile, the bile acids are coupled in amide linkage to glycine and taurine as *glycocholic* and *taurocholic* acids.

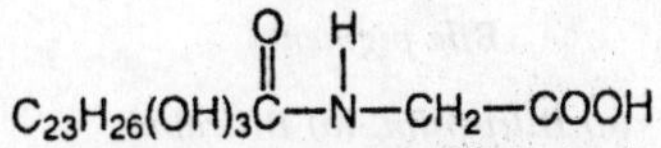

Glycocholic acid (Cholylglycine)

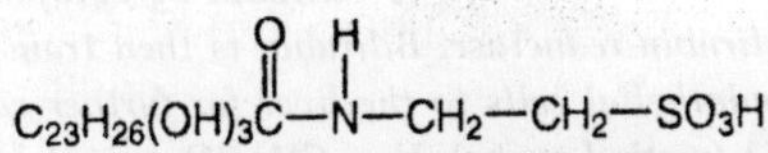

Taurocholic acid (Cholyltaurine)

At the pH of bile (7.3 to 7.7) *glycocholate* and *taurocholate* exist as anions, but they do not contribute to the osmotic pressure of the bile. The role of bile salts in the digestion of fats is secondary to its important function of enhancing the absorption of digested fats by the intestinal villi. Bile salts reduce the surface tension of the absorbing epithelium, increase their permeability and thus facilitate absorption. This is known as *hydrotropic action*. The fats can be easily digested even in the absence of bile. However, it is quite interesting that in the absence of bile, the products of fat-digestion and other fat-soluble substances are not absorbed, but are eliminated with the faeces.

The *bile pigments,* biliverdin and bilirubin are derived from degradation of haemoglobin in liver cells and give the bile its characteristic colour. In humans, *bilirubin* is the predominant pigment, so that human bile is golden yellow. Normally, bilirubin is converted in the intestine into more soluble *urobilinogen* and this pigment, together with other breakdown products, gives faeces its brown colour.

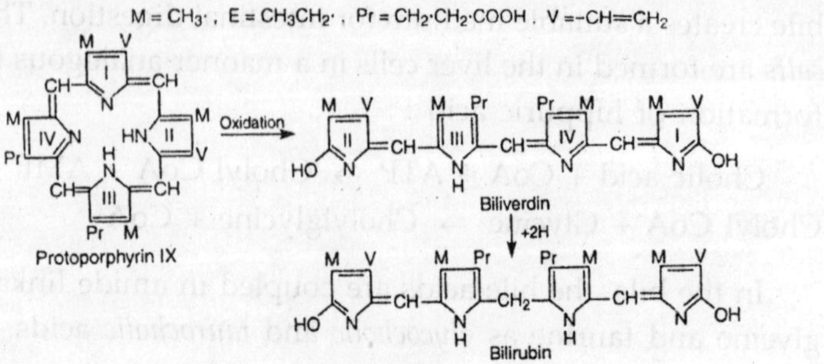

Bile pigments

(a) Biliverdin, (b) Bilirubin.

Biliverdin is oxidized to bilirubin by cytoplasmic NADPH-bilirubin reductase. Bilirubin is then transported from reticuloendothelial cells to the liver for further catabolism. M=—CH3 (methyl group), V=—CH=CH_2 (vinyl group), and P=—CH_2—CH_2—COOH (propionic acid group) on the pyrrole rings.

Digestion in Large Intestine

The colon bacteria secrete the enzymes that work upon proteins and cellose of plants. These enzymes are not very important in man, but in herbivores, they digest cellulose. The material that reaches the large intestine has most of its nutrients already taken away from it.

The principal enzymes of the digestive tract and the substances they hydrolyse are given in Table. The physiology of mammalian digestion is summarized in Fig.

Hormonal Control of Digestive Secretions : The action of the digestive glands is controlled by the nervous system and by hormones. Salivary glands are controlled entirely by the nervous system and may also be influenced by the higher centres of brain, such as thinking about or seeing the food. The flow of gastric juice is regulated partly by a nervous mechanism and partly by the action of the hormone *gastrin,* which is produced in the mucosa cells of the stomach.

Summary of Enzymatic Hydrolysis of the Food Materials in Humans

S. No.	Name of digestive juice	Name of gland secreting it	Region of action	Optimum pH	Substrate	Enzyme	End product
1.	Saliva	Salivary gland	Buccal cavity	about 7 (neutral or slightly alkaline)	starch	Salivary amylase	maltose
2.	Gastric juice	Gastric gland	Stomach	2.0 (acidic)	proteins	(a) Pepsin	peptides
					caseinogen	(b) Rennin	casein
					fat	(c) Gastric lipase	glycerol and fatty acids
3.	Pancreatic juice	Cells of exocrine pancreas	Small intestine	7-8 (alkaline)	proteins	(a) Trypsin	peptides and free
					proteins	(b) Chymotrypsin	amino acids
					peptides	(c) Caroxypeptidase	free amino acids
					starch	(d) Amylase or amylopsin	maltose
					fats	(e) Pancreatic lipase or steapsin	glycerol and fatty acids
					maltose	(f) maltase	glucose
					RNA	(g) ribonuclease	nucleotides
4.	Intestinal juice (Succus entericus)	Intestinal glands	Small intestine	7-8 (alkaline)	trypsinogen	(a) enteropeptidase	trypsin
					peptones and proteoses	(b) erepsin	amino acids
					maltose	(c) maltase	glucose
					sucrose	(d) sucrase	glucose and fructose
					lactose	(e) lactase	glucose and galactose
					peptides	(f) peptidases	amino acids
					fats	(g) lipase	fatty acids and glycerol
					DNA and RNA	(h) nucleases	nucleotides, nucleosides and bases.

Summary of Hormonal Factors Controlling the Flow of Digestive Juices.

S. No.	*Name of hormone*	*Secreted by*	*Place of action*	*Function*	*Other factors affecting the secretion of the juice*
1.	Gastrin	Stomach into the bloodstream	Gastric glands	Induces the secretion of gastric juice by gastric glands	Neural (simple and conditioned reflex)
2.	Secretin	Small intestine into the blood-stream.	Cells of exocrine pancreas	Stimulates the secretion of large amount of pancreatic juice low in digestive enzymes.	Neural (simple reflex)
3.	Pancreozymin	—do—	—do—	Stimulates the secretion of pancreatic juice rich in digestive enzymes.	
4.	Enterocrinin	—do—	Intestinal glands	Enhances the secretion of intestinal juice.	
5.	Duocrinin	—do—	—do—	—do—	
6.	Cholecvstokinin	—do—	Gallbladder	Contraction and emptying of gall bladder.	Neural (simple reflex)

The hormones *secretin* and *pancreozymin* stimulate the pancreas for secreting the pancreatic juice, but nervous impulses may also play a minor role. The secretion of intestinal juice is influenced by two specific hormones called *enterocrinin* and *duocrinin*, together with the action of the intrinsic nerves of the intestinal wall. During digestion, the gall bladder is emptied as a result of the action of the hormone *cholecystokinin*, which is secreted by the wall of the small intestine. The most effective stimuli for the liberation of cholecystokinin are fats and meat extracts. A summary of the hormonal factors controlling the secretion of the digestive juices is given in Table.

Absorption

It is the process by which the end products of digestion pass through the intestinal epithelium and enter the bloodstream. In humans, there is little absorption in the stomach which can absorb water, alcohol and small amounts of mineral salts. Small intestine is mainly responsible for major absorption, since the intestinal villi contain the absorptive epithelial cells and a network of blood and lymph capillaries (Fig.) which readily pick up the digested materials.

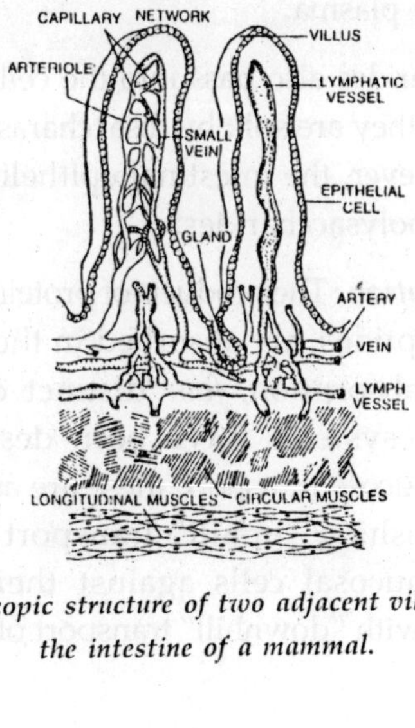

Microscopic structure of two adjacent villi from the intestine of a mammal.

Carbohydrate Absorption : The greatest amount of carbohydrate is absorbed as monosaccharides. Both pentoses and hexoses diffuse easily through the intestinal wall. Passive diffusion is perhaps the only mechanism of uptake for several monosaccharides normally present in the food such as fructose, mannose, and most pentoses. The uptake of glucose and galactose by the intestinal epithelial cells is aided by active transport.

The driving force for this active transport is provided by the Na^+, K^+-ATPase at the basolateral membrane of the epithelial cell, which pumps Na^+ out of the cell, thus maintaining the Na^+ gradient. As Na^+ moves into the cell down its concentration gradient, the coupled transport of monosaccharide against its concentration gradient is able to occur. The carrier is an integral membrane protein that binds and transports two Na^+ ions for each sugar molecule. Its glucose site, but not its Na^+ site, can be blocked by the glycoside phlorizin. Inhibitors of the Na^+, K^+-ATPase system such as ovabain also block glucose absorption because of the resultant inability of the epithelial cell to transfer Na^+ from its serosal side to the plasma.

Some disaccharides also pass into the cells of the intestinal epithelium where they are split by disaccharases such as lactase and maltase. However, the intestinal epithelium is practically impermeable to polysaccharides.

Protein Absorption : The products of protein digestion, amino acids and oligopeptides, are absorbed in the small intestine. For amino acid absorption, *four* distinct carrier-mediated active transport systems have been described. Like the mechanisms for glucose transport, these are also Na^+ symport systems accomplishing "uphill" transport of the L-amino acids into the mucosal cells against their concentration gradients, along with "downhill" transport of Na^+ into the cell.

The energy for this transport comes from Na^+, K^+- ATPase. The four systems are as follows :

(a) *Transport System for Neutral Amino Acids :* The amino acids transported by this system are Alanine, Glycine, Serine, Threonine, Valine, Leucine, Isoleucine, Phenylalanine, Tyrosine, Tryptophan, Aspartate, Histidine, Cysteine, Methionine and Citrulline.

(b) *Transport System for Dibasic (diamino) Amino Acids :* There appears to be two distinct pathways for transport of dibasic amino acids. One transports Lysine, Arginine, Ornithine, and Cystine and the other transports Lysine, Arginine, and Ornithine but not Cystine.

(c) *Transport System for Dicarboxylic (acidic) Amino Acids :* This transports Aspartic acid and Glutamic acid.

(d) *Transport System for Glycine and Imino Acids :* This transports Glycine, Proline, and Hydroxyproline.

Some amino acids such as glycine have affinity for more than one of the transport systems. For any given transport system, the amino acids mentioned under these systems compete for the carrier binding sites. Besides amino acids, oligopeptides can also be transported across the intestinal epithelial cells by distinct mechanisms. At least two distinct pathways for transport of small peptides are known. One actively transports di- and tripeptides and appears to be a Na^+ symport. The transported peptides bypass the brush border peptidases and are then hydrolyzed by cytoplasmic peptidases. Another pathway utilized for larger peptides involves initial hydrolysis by brush border peptidases followed by carrier-mediated transport of the released amino acids. Although amino acids are more rapidly absorbed in the proximal small intestine, peptidases are well absorbed from both proximal and distal parts. Amino acids present in the mucosal cells diffuse into the portal blood and then to the liver.

***Fat Absorption* :** The mechanism of fat absorption is still a matter of discussion. There has been much debate about whether unhydrolyzed fat can be absorbed or whether partial, or complete hydrolysis (lipolysis) is necessary. However, now it is known that regardless of the form in which fat is transferred from the lumen of the intestine into the epithelial cells, it is present as triglyceride when it leaves the cells to enter the lymphatic vessels.

Recent experiments have shown that 25—60% of the fat appears to be fully hydrolyzed to free fatty acids before absorption. The greater part of the remaining fat seems to be absorbed as monoglyceride, whereas only a little of fat is absorbed as di- and triglycerides. Electron microscopy has suggested that ingested fat may be taken up by epithelial cells in the form of microdroplets by the process of pinocytosis or phagocytosis. Diffusion appears to be the usual mechanism of uptake for molecularly dispersed glycerides or free fatty acids. The dispersion of fats and their digestive products appears to be aided by the bile salts, which form water-soluble complexes with the fatty acids. Uptake by diffusion appears to be further supplemented by the solubility of the free acids in the cell membranes.

The crucial role of bile salts in promoting the absorption of fatty acids and monoacylglycerols relates to their ability to form mixed *micelles* with these products (Fig.). These micelles are 40 to 60 Å in diameter. Water insoluble fatty acids and monoacylglycerols resulting from lipase action are solubilized within the micelle with their polar head groups facing outward and their hydrophobic hydrocarbon chains within the centre of the micelle. Mixed micelles of bile salts, fatty acids, and monoacylglycerols form spontaneously whenever the critical micellar concentration of the bile salts is exceeded.

These micelles also contain the lipid-soluble vitamins (A, D, E, and K), cholesterol and phosphatidylcholine. Because tri- and diacylglycerols are so hydrophobic, they remain in the oil phase of the intestinal contents. Subsequent to lipase hydrolysis, the released fatty acids and monoacylglycerols enter the aqueous phase via the process of solubilization in micelles. The concentration of these substances in the micelles is 1000 times greater than their concentration in the aqueous phase.

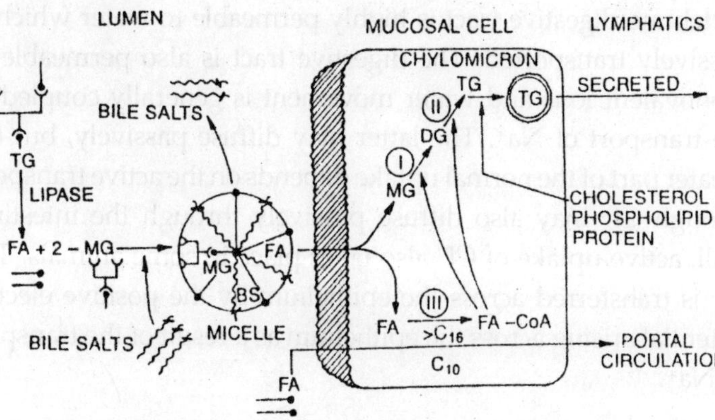

Schematic representation of digestion and absorption of dietary lipid. Roman numerals indicate enzymes catalyzing various reactions. I monoacylglycerol acyltransferase, II diacylglycerol acyltransferase, III Acyl CoA synthetase. BS bile salt C_{10}, C_{16} fatty acid, chain length, DG diacylglycerol, FA fatty acid, MG monoacylgylcerol, TG Triacylgylcerol.

Thus, micelles markedly increase the rate of delivery of the fatty acids and monoacylglycerols to the intestinal mucosa, which represents the absorptive surface. The fatty acids, monoacylglycerols and fat-soluble vitamins leave the micelles and, being lipid-soluble, passively diffuse across the membranes of the epithelial cells down their concentration gradients. This process of absorption is largely completed in the upper jejunum.

The products of the digestion of medium chain triacylglycerols (C_8 to C_{12}) are water soluble. Hence, they do not require micellar solubilization and are directly absorbed into the intestinal cell. Similarly, the water-soluble glycerol is also directly absorbed. Once within the intestinal mucosal cell, the fate of the fatty acids is determined in large part by their chain length. Long chain fatty acids, which are the main component of the dietary lipid, are re-esterified to form triglycerols.

Water and Electrolyte Absorption : It is known that the vertebrate digestive tract is highly permeable to water which is passively transported. The digestive tract is also permeable to monovalent ions and water movement is generally coupled to the transport of Na^+. The latter may diffuse passively, but the greater part of the normal uptake depends on the active transport. Though Cl^- may also diffuse passively through the intestinal wall, active uptake of Cl^- also takes place in some animals. The Cl^- is transferred across the epithelium by the positive electric potential arising across the epithelium as a result of the transport of Na^+.

The intestine is rather impermeable to di- and trivalent ions. However, the absorption of Ca^{2+}, Fe^{2+}, and Fe^{3+}, depends on the specific active mechanisms.

Mechanism of Absorption

The mechanism of absorption has been explained on the basis of several physico-chemical principles. Of them, *diffusion* is the most important. The concentration of the end products of digestion is much higher in the intestine than in the blood. This difference initiates diffusion currents from the lumen of the intestine into the bloodstream and thus helps in absorption.

It has been established that the *phenomenon of active transport* plays a fading role in the process of absorption. The active transport mechanism involves movement of materials from the intestine to the blood and lymph of villi against a concentration gradient and needs energy. Since the intestinal wall has the ability to transport many substances actively, they can be removed from the intestine even though they may be present in the blood in a higher concentration.

Interactions may also occur between the active transport of different molecules. For example, the active transport of glucose depends upon the simultaneous transport of Na^+ across the intestinal epithelium. However, interference has also been observed between the active transport of glucose and a number of amino acids that inhibit the transport of glucose.

According to *Moog* (1981), the inner surface of the intestine is active both in *breaking down* and in *absorbing* nutrients. The structure of the *absorptive* cell (Fig.) of the intestinal lining reflects its specialized

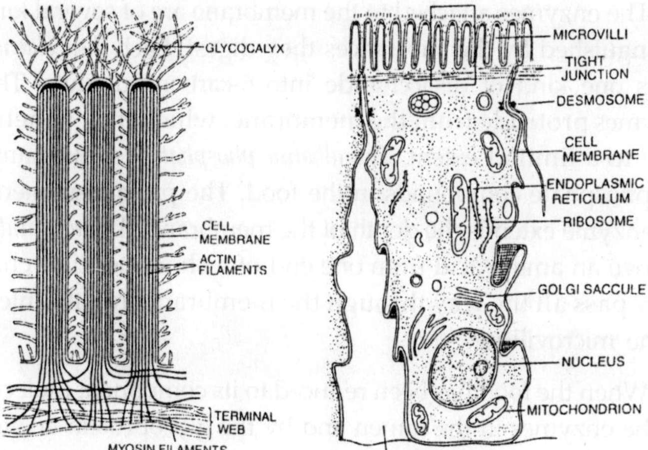

Structure of the absorptive epithelial cell of the intestinal lining with brush border magnified.

function in digestion. The most striking feature of the cell is the *brush border* which is made up of rows of minute projections called *microvilli* which are about a micrometre long, and they are packed at a density of 200,000 per mm^2 in the human jejunum. They increase the surface area of the small intestine by a factor of about 20. In the interior of each microvillus is a core of protein fibres (actin filaments). The fibres from all the microvilli in each absorptive cell run down to a layer of fibres called the terminal web.

The outer membrane of each microvillus is covered by a *glycocalyx* (Fig.), a carbohydrate coat thicker than that of the most cell membranes. The glycocalyx extends from the tip of the microvillus into the intestinal lumen. It is now known that some of the glycocalyx fibres are parts of the digestive enzyme molecules embedded in the membrane of the microvilli. The enzymes are *glycoproteins,* made up of a protein with several attached carbohydrate chains; the carbohydrate portion extending into the lumen.

The enzymes attached to the membrane are of several kinds, distinguished by the substances they digest. Each *disaccharidase* splits one kind of disaccharide into 6-carbon subunits. These enzymes protrude from the membrane, which they penetrate only to a limited extent. The *alkaline phosphatase* splits many of the phosphate compounds in the food. The protein segment of the enzyme extends the depth of the membrane. *Aminopeptidases* remove an amino acid from one end of a short peptide chain. They pass all the way through the membrane into the interior of the microvillus.

When the food has been reduced to its component molecules by the enzymes in the lumen and by the glycoprotein enzymes attached to the microvillus membrane, the nutrients must be absorbed into the bloodstream. It is well known that the starch, the main source of carbohydrate in most human diets, is reduced to maltose by *amylase* in the mouth and in the lumen.

Some of the amylase molecules may be trapped in glycocalyx fibres along with other pancreatic enzymes. As mentioned above, the maltase attached to the brush-border membrane splits each molecule of maltose into two molecules of glucose. With the help of a carrier (a molecule of maltose after splitting the disaccharide might serve as a carrier for the 6-carbon sugars) these glucose molecules move into the microvillus. However, it is now known that the maltase on the membrane is capable of splitting far more maltose than this transport system could carry. Some of the liberated glucose molecules are released into the lumen from where they may return to the surface of a villus. It is assumed that a second transport system then carries glucose molecules across the membrane. In this system the movement of glucose molecules is coupled to the transport of sodium ions across the membrane in the same direction. The parallel flow of Na^+ ions provides the energy needed for the accumulation of glucose beyond the concentration present in the lumen.

The uptake of amino acids appears to require four active transport systems that are quite independent of one another. These systems correspond to the four classes of the amino acids. The 15 *neutral amino acids* (the largest class) are transported rapidly but at rates that vary with the affinity of the amino acid for the carrier. Thus, all amino acids with similar chemical structure compete for entry by means of the same transport system.

The three *dibasic amino acids*, which have two amino groups, also compete among themselves for a common transport site. Glycine, proline and hydroxyproline have an affinity for a third carrier. Glutamic acid and aspartic acid also have their own system. Whether or not the fourth transport system moves amino acids into the cell against a concentration gradient is difficult to say, because these amino acids are immediately converted into glutamine and asparagine. Hence glutamic acid and aspartic acid do not accumulate in the cell. However, the movement of amino acids in all the four ways (systems) requires energy and is coupled with a parallel flow of Na^+ ions.

In recent years, the picture of protein absorption has been complicated further and it is now evident that dipeptides and tripeptides can also proceed directly into the absorptive cell. Once they are across the membrane, they are reduced to amino acids by the action of peptidases in the cytoplasm.

Recent work in physiology has shown that the lining of the small intestine is active both in breaking down and in absorbing nutrients. The membrane of the lining cells is equipped with diverse array of transport systems. When digestion is complete these carriers transport simple sugars, amino acids and small peptides into the cytoplasm of the cells from where the nutrients are absorbed into the blood.

Elimination

Undigested materials are eliminated from the lower part of the intestine in the form of faeces. The characteristic brown colour of the faeces is due to the excretion of bile pigments from the liver.

Assimilation or Ultimate Fate of the Absorbed Materials : Absorbed amino acids and glucose are carried by the hepatic portal system to the liver, where they are stored, changed into other forms and released to the blood. Many of the amino acids are deaminized in the liver by the removal of the amino group (NH_2), which then combines with carbon dioxide to form urea CO $(NH_2)_2$, a waste product of urine. Remaining amino acids are converted into fat or sugar for energy purposes. Other amino acids are released by the liver to the cells of the body to repair or replace living protoplasm.

The glucose is converted to glycogen (animal starch) in the liver, where it is stored to be released (as glucose) to the blood for the maintenance of the glucose level (0.1%). Some glucose combines with other substances to form a basic part of protoplasm, and some is also stored in the muscles as glycogen. Glucose is one of the most available sources of energy for muscular work and heat production.

The fat that enters the bloodstream, from the thoracic duct is changed into fat characteristic of animal's body by rearrangements of the fatty acids. Some fats in the form of lipids enter into the structure of protoplasm, especially at cell surfaces, where they help to form the nuclear and plasma membranes. Excess fat is stored in adipose tissues which are located in the connective tissues between muscles and skin, in mesenteries and around various organs.

Protection against Self-digestion

The efficiency of digestive enzymes raises an important problem, *i.e.,* what prevents them from digesting the cells that produce them, or the lining of the stomach and intestine. The answer is that it is not sufficient simply to manufacture the potent digestive enzymes. But they must in addition be prevented from exercising their powers of protein digestion until the appropriate time and place. Pepsin and trypsin are not elaborated as such in the gland cells of stomach and pancreas respectively. Instead, they are first secreted as inactive molecules of *pepsinogen* and *trypsinogen.* When they reach the stomach which has low pH, or the alkaline contents of the small intestine, they are converted into active form, *pepsin* and *trypsin.* A little active pepsin or trypsin already present accelerates this change and the activation therefore proceeds at a rapid rate once the pepsinogen or the trypsinogen reaches the place where it is needed. Thus, active enzymes work only on the food molecules (substrates) and not on the living cells of the gut epithelium.

Further protection is provided by the large amount of mucus secreted by the cells that line the digestive tract. The mucous forms an effective barrier against the active digestive enzymes.

Malfunction of Digestive System

Peptic Ulcer : There may be several causes and symptoms of malfunctioning of the digestive system. Malfunctioning may result into peptic ulcer :

A peptic ulcer may be caused in either of two ways :

(i) excess secretion of hydrochloric acid and pepsin by the gastric mucosa, or

(ii) diminished ability of the gastroduodenal mucosal barrier to protect against the digestive properties of the acid-pepsin complex.

Among specific causes of peptic ulcer in humans, bacterial infection by *Helieobacter pylori* plays an important role. At least 75 per cent of peptic ulcer patients have been found to have chronic infection of the gastic mucosa and duodenal mucosa by this bacterium. It is capable of penetrating the mucosal barrier both by virtue of its physical capability to burrow through the barrier and by releasing digestive enzymes that liquefy the barrier. As a result, the strong acidic digestive juices of the stomach can penetrate into the underlying epithalium and digest the epithelial cells. This leads to peptic ulceration.

In addition to excess secretion of gastric juices and bacterial infection, other factors that predispose to ulcers are smoking, alcohol and aspirin.

The common sites of peptic ulcer are the first part of the duodenum *(duodenal ulcer)* and in the stomach *(gastric ulcer)*, usually on the lesser curvature a few inches from the pyloric sphincter.

Persons having *gastric ulcer* may exhibit anxiety or other emotional states which by stimulating the vagal mechanism lead to intense congestion and hypersecretion. Actual haemorrhage may take place and the gastric juice may digest and so further damage any abnormal area.

In patients with *duodenal ulcer* there is overactivity of gastric vagi. As a result, the stomach is hypermotile and empties rapidly, a large volume of highly acid juice is secreted which is imperfectly neutralised. It is thought that the discharge of the very acid juice into the duodenum produces local damage.

The pain of the *peptic ulcer* is probably due mainly to the action of acid or other irritants on a hypersensitive region of the mucous membrane. The pain generally occurs when gastric acidity reaches a characteristic threshold level, *e.g.*, pH 1.5 or lower levels of acidity. The ingestion of food, which decreases gastric acidity, relieves the pain. Vomitting, which removes acid fluid from the stomach, also relieves the pain. In both types of peptic ulcer, pain is relieved by *antacids*.

Because vagal overaction may be an important causal factor in peptic ulcer, *vagotomy* may be done in some cases. In this operation both vagus nerves that supply parasympathetic stimulation to the gastric glands are cut, usually where they lie on the surface of the lower part of the oesophagus. This temporarly blocks almost all secretion of acid and pepsin and often cures the ulcer within one week after the operation.

The ulcer patients are also treated effectively by the use of *antibiotics* such as tetracycline along with other agents to kill the infectious bacteria, and by the administration of an acid-suppressant drug, especially *ranitidine*.

Physiology of Digestion in Invertebrates : Invertebrates have almost the same food materials to digest as vertebrates and thus, they have proteases, lipases, amylases and other hydrolytic enzymes. However, the structure of the digestive system is different, and there is a great variation in the details of the digestive processes. One characteristic difference is that invertebrates have no proteolytic enzymes, that act in highly acidic solution, as does the pepsin of vertebrates. It is possible that the evolution of the peptic digestion is associated with the ingestion of large prey, where skeletal material is more easily disintegrated in a strong acid. Thus, pepsin and hydrochloric acid are found throughout all higher vertebrate classes from fish to man.

In other respects, invertebrate digestive enzymes are similar to the vertebrate digestive enzymes, although some invertebrates can easily digest substances indigestible to vertebrates. For example, the clothes moth can digest hair and wool, and cellulose can also be digested by many invertebrates. Some of them have cellulases, but others depend on microbes living in their digestive tracts for cellulose digestion.

Symbiotic Digestion

This is a mode of digestion carried out by the microorganisms and protozoans living in the digestive tracts of some animals as symbionts. These microbes act upon certain materials that cannot be hydrolysed by the enzymes of the animal concerned and change them into digestible substances. The digestion of cellulose in termites and mammals, and the wax-digestion in honey guides (a bird) are some important examples of symbiotic digestion.

In mammals, symbiotic digestion may be either pregastric or postgastric. The former takes place in ruminates as well as in other animals such as the camel and Ilama, and in the Quokka *(Setonix branchyurus)* and other macropode marsupials. No digestive enzymes are secreted by the wall of the rumen and digestion occurs practically by means of bacteria and ciliates. Enzymes called hydrolases, secreted by the microorganisms carry out the initial digestion of food. However, the sugars so produced are largely utilized by the microorganisms, themselves. In anaerobic environment these sugars are degraded by fermentation resulting in the formation of volatile fatty acids like acetic acid, propionic acid, and butyric acid. These fatty acids are utilized by the host itself. The enzymes secreted by the microorganisms include amylase and oligosaccharases in addition to glycosidases.

In ruminant digestion, the proteins of the food are split by proteinases secreted by the microorganisms. Though amino acids may be absorbed through the wall of the rumen, their major part is used by the microorganisms for growth. The microorganisms themselves eventually pass from the rumen to the stomach proper in which they are utilized. Thus microorganisms represent the most important source of protein to the host. The rumen microbes are also able to utilize urea and ammonia for protein synthesis. The urea produced in the liver is returned to the rumen by diffusion from the blood and in the saliva and can be reutilized for protein synthesis by microorganisms. As the proteins are scanty in the diet, this capacity is of great importance in protein economy of the ruminant. In addition to the above advantages, microorganisms also synthesize many vitamins which can be utilized by the host.

Accesory Organs

In addition to the teeth, tongue and salivary glands, which are structures accesory to the digestive system, two abdominal glands are of prime importance in the digestive process. These are : (a) the *liver* and (b) the *pancreas.*

The Liver

The liver is the largest gland in the body. Its upper and anterior surfaces are smooth and curved to fit the under surface of the diaphragm; the posterior surface is irregular in outline. It consists of 3 lobes in frog: *right, left and median;* 5 in rabbit: *left lateral, left central spigelian, right central* and *caudate;* 4 in man : *right, left, quadrats and caudate lobe.* These are surrounded by a thick *capsule,* mostly overlaid with reflected peritoneum.

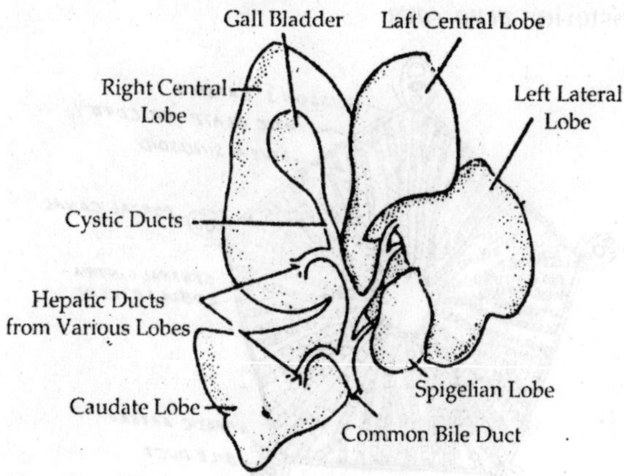

Liver of Rabbit

Structure of Liver : The liver is the largest organ in the body, contributing about 1/50 of the total body weight, or about 1.4 kg in the average adult human. The functional unit of the liver is the *liver lobule* which is a cylindrical structure 0.8 to 2 mm in diameter and several millimeters in length.

Classic Hepatic Lobule

The parenchyma in the interior of liver, is subdivided into myriads of small lobules. Each lobule is incompletely isolated by connective tissue septum named *Glissoris Capsule.* This capsule is absent around liver lobules of man. Each lobular unit consists of two chief components :

(a) *Parenchyma.* It is composed of many *hepatic cellular plates* that radiate from the central vein like spokes in a wheel. Each hepatic plate is usually two cells thickened between the adjacent cells lie small *bile canaliculi* that empty into *Hering's canals* walled by cuboidal epithelium. These canals lead into *bile ducts* in the fibrous septa separating the adjacent liver lobules.

The liver lobule is constructed around a *central vein* that empties into the hepatic veins and then into the posterior *vena cava.*

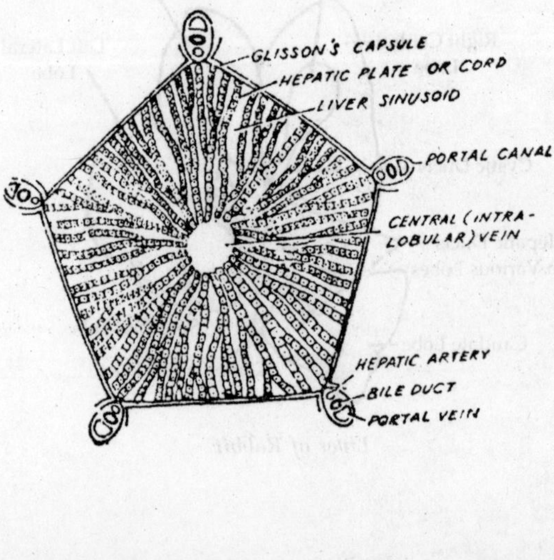

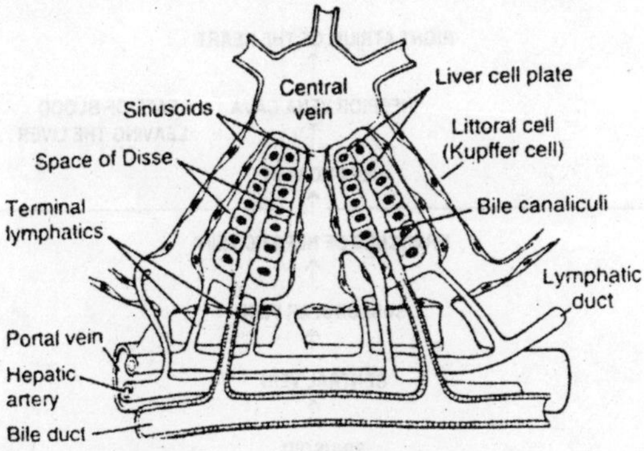

Basic Structure of a liver lobule, showing the hepatic cellular plates, the blood vessels, the bile-collecing system and the lymph flow system composed of the spaces of Disse and the interlobular lymphatics.

(b) *Sinusoids :* The hepatic plates are separated by hepatic sinusoids that converge radially into the *central vein* in their radial course, they tunnel the parenchyma into plate-like cords. Such channels communicate with both the central vein and vessels at the periphery. They receive blood from *hepatic artery* (25%) and *portal vein* (75%) at the periphery of the lobule and discharge it into the central vein in the axis of the lobule. Each central vein connects at right angles with a *sublobular vein* which is a solitary collecting vessel coursing along the base of a lobule Sublobular veins are tributary to branches of the *hepatic veins* proper. The latter open into the *postcaval* or inferior vena cava.

They are intensely phagocytic and belong to the group of fixed macrophagus. The Kupffer cells devour bacteria, worn-out blood cells and foreign particles in the hepatic sinus blood. These cells efficiently cleanse blood as it passes through the sinuses. When a bacterium comes into momentary contact with a Kupffer cell, it immediately passes inwards through the well of the Kupffer cell to become permanently lodged therein until it gets digested.

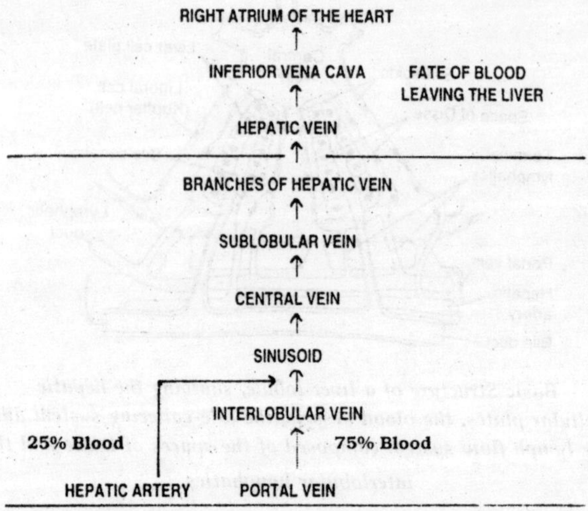

Scheme of blood flow through the liver

Between the endothelial cells of the sinusoids and the hepatic cells are present narrow tissue spaces called the *spaces of Disse*. The millions of these spaces in turn connect with lymphatic vessels in the interlobular septa. The extreme permeability of the liver sinusoid epithelium allows large quantities of lymph to form in the spaces of Disse. Therefore, about 1/2 of all the lymph formed in the body under resting conditions arises in the liver.

Portal Canals

Connective tissue at the edges of a lobule, constitutes the so-called portal canals. Within each canal occur the conspicious components of the hepatic triad. It comprises a branch of an *hepatic artery*, *portal vein* and *bile duct*. The portal canals are "gateways" through which blood reaches the liver.

The functional components of a portal canal are as follows:

(a) *Portal-Vein* : It conveys venous blood, from the stomach, spleen and intestines to the liver. This blood is poor in oxygen but rich in nourishment. Portal vein is the largest component of hepatic triad, but it is very thin-walled. Its smallest branches lie between the lobules and are called *interlobular veins*. These breakdown into precapillaries which connect directly with intralobular sinusoids.

Venous blood of portal veins is the primary supply (75 percent) of the hepatic lobules.

(b) *Hepatic Artery* : Although rather thick walled, it is usually the smallest component.

These vessels supply about 25 per cent of the total blood to hepatic lobules.

(c) *Bile Duct* : Its size is intermediate between that of the two blood vessels. It carries bile to the hepatic ducts.

Several small hepatic ducts bringing bile from different lobes of the liver are joined by a cystic duct from the gall bladder, thus forming a large common bile duct opening into the duodenum. The gall bladder acts as a reservoir for the storage of bile which, after leaving the liver by the hepatic duct, passes up the cystic duct to the interior of the gall bladder where a remains until it is required for the purpose of digestion. After a meal, especially if it contains fat, the gall bladder contracts and expels the bile via the cystic duct and common bile duct into the duodenum. During its stay in the gall bladder, the bile is concentrated by the absorption of water.

The hepatic lobule is quite unlike lobules of ordinary glands. The axis of a liver lobule is an endothelium-lined tube, the central vein instead of the customary duct. This type of lobulation is an adaptation of certain activities peculiar to liver, like glycogenesis etc.

Portal Lobule

A different kind of Lobule, the portal lobule is recognized in the liver with reference to *bile secretion.* This unit is formed from parts of 3 hepatic lobules that adjoin a portal canal. It is the area drained by an interlobular bile duct in a portal canal. The functional boundary of such a portal lobule extends from one central vein to another. The bile duct, located in the common portal canal (where the edges of 3 hepatic lobules meet), forms axis of such a portal lobule.

The portal lobule is a *functional unit* which is used in connection with liver physiology and pathology.

Functions of Liver

Liver, the largest gland of vertebrate body, is an essential organ, which performs many functions :

Secretion : It secretes *bile* which is a complex watery fluid containing bile salts (Na taurocholate and glycocholate), bile pigments (biliverdin and bilirubin), cholesterol, mucin, lecithin and fats etc. The bile aids in intestinal digestion as it breaks and emulsifies the fat, prevents purification of food by checking the growth of bacteria, makes the chyme better suited for pancreatic digestion by neutralizing the acid in it, and helps in the absorption of fat from the intestine.

Excretion : In the liver, haemoglobin of the worn out erythrocytes breaks down to bile pigments *bilirubin* and *biliverdin*. The bile pigments are converted in the bowel into *stercobilin* which colours the faeces but, apart from this, are waste products having no other function.

Glycogenesis : Excess quantities of carbohydrates (glucose) are converted to glycogen in the presence of *insulin* in the liver cells, and stored therein.

Glycogenolysis : Glycogen is a reserve food material which is changed into glucose and released into the blood at concentrations maintained constant by the liver. In this way, blood-sugar level is maintained under diverse dietary conditions.

Gluconeogenesis : Under abnormal conditions, liver can convert proteins and fats into glucose by complex chemical reactions. Formation of this "new sugar" *i.e.*, from non-carbohydrate sources, is called gluconeogenesis.

Lipogenesis : If the level of blood-glucose rises beyond normal even after glycogenesis and catabolism, the excess glucose is converted into fat and stored in the liver. The process is termed lipogenesis.

Transamination and Deamination : Amino-acids resulting from protein digestion finally come into the liver from the intestines. They are partly released into the blood for distribution and *protein synthesis*, partly *transaminated* into the other amino-acids and *deaminated*. Any resulting keto-acids are converted into carbohydrates or fats and the free amino-groups appear as ammonia. This is excreted as such *(e.g.*, aquatic animals) or after prior conversion to urea *(e.g.*. amphibians, mammals) or uric acid *(e.g.*, insects and birds).

Hemopoiesis : In the embryo, red blood cells are manufactured by the liver. In the adult, liver stores inorganic salts of iron, copper and vitamin B_{12} (anti-anaemic factor) and thus helps in the formation of red cells and haemoglobin.

Store-house of Blood : Liver functions as a store-house *for* blood and regulates blood-volume. Its normal blood volume, including both in the hepatic veins and that in the hepatic sinuses, is 450 ml, or almost 10% of the body's total blood volume.

Blood Clotting : *Fibrinogen, Prothrombin* and certain other blood coagulation factors are formed in the liver which are instrumental in blood-clotting. *Heparin* is an intravascular anticoagulant that is stored in the liver. It originates in mast cells which are abundant in the liver, among other sites.

Production of Plasma Proteins : The plasma proteins serum albumin and serum globulin are synthesized by the liver from the amino-acids derived from the protein in the diet.

Synthesis and Storage of Vitamins : Liver synthesizes vitamin A from the provitamins A (carotenoid pigments). Liver cells also store fat-soluble vitamins A, D, K and E. Besides, it is the principal storage organ for vitamin B_{12}.

Detoxication : It is the process by which toxic substances are rapidly made extractable through different biochemical changes. The liver is the site of detoxication of different toxic substances either produced in the body or taken alongwith food. This is done by the process of *oxidation, hydrolysis, reduction* and *conjugation*. Many drugs like *phenylbutazone, Pethidine, chloromycetin* etc. are also made exretable by the liver enzymes.

Alcohol Metabolism : Liver is the main site of alcohol metabolism. By various enzymes in the liver, alcohol is first catabolised to acetaldehyde which is converted into acetyle CoA. The latter may be oxidised to CO_2 and H_2O or converted to other biochemical compounds including fatty acids through TCA cycle.

The direct effect of alcohol may be alcoholic fatty liver which results from increased fatty acid synthesis.

Desaturation of Fats : Fats are stored in the body in a saturated from *i.e.,* they cannot take any more hydrogen into their composition). Before the saturated fats can be used by the tissues of the body, they are conveyed to the liver which converts them into unsaturated form (by the removal of hydrogen). The unsaturated fats are then used by the tissues to provide energy.

Heat Production : A large number of chemical processes are carried out by the liver, that involve the production of great deal of heat. It is the main heat producing organ of the body.

Phagocytosis : Kupffer cells in the liver sinusoids phagocytose and remove bacteria, worm-out blood elements and foreign particles.

The Pancreas

The pancreas is a pale yellow gland which is found in the region of the junction between the stomach and the duodenum. It is a heterocrine gland which performs both *exo*—as well as *endocrin* functions.

***Structure* :** The pancreas is a rather diffuse gland which is a mixture of two histologically and functionally separate tissues. The bulk of the gland is exocrine in function, and is drained by the pancreatic duct that opens into the duodenum. Scattered among the exocrine cells are patches of tissue named Islets of Langerhans (1869) after their discover, and these consist of endocrine cell to the blood. Each islet is an epithelial mass, tunneled by labyrinthine capillaries.

3 types of cells can be distinguished in Islets on the basis of solubility, staining etc.

(i) *Alpha cells,* or A-cells, are fairly numerous in most islets. Their granules are soluble in water but not in alcohol.

(ii) *Beta cells,* or B-cells are smaller and usually much more numerous. Their granules are coarser but alcohol soluble.

(iii) *Delta cells* or D-cells are the rarest. It is not definite whether they are a separate cell-type or a developmental stage.

***Functions* :** The pancreas is a gland having two different types of secretions :

(1) An Internal Secretion from the Islets of Langerhans, which is absorbed directly into the blood. There are 4 hormones present in this secretion :

(a) *Insulin,* secreted by the β-cells. The function of insulin is to convert excess blood sugar (glucose) into glycogen that is stored in the liver.

(b) *Glycagon,* secreted by the α -cells. This hormone converts liver glycogen to glucose.

(c) *Gāstrin,* secreted by D-cells. It is similar to the hormone produced by the stomach, but is very small in amount.

(2) An External Secretion (pancreatic juice), which leaves the gland by the pancreatic duct. The external secretion is an important digestive juice and contains the following enzymes:

(a) *Amylase,* which converts all starches into maltose.

(b) *Trypsin,* which converts peptones into amino-acids.

(c) *Lipase,* which splits fats into fatty acids and glycerol.

4

Absorption of Food

Digestion is a process by which food substances are altered *physically* and *chemically*, so that they are reduced to simple assimilable forms. The process is divided into two main parts:

Mechanical Digestion : The phase of digestion comprises *liquifying* of food by the digestive juices. *mastication, swallowing,* and thereafter onward movement through the tract by *peristalsis.* It is a special method of muscular contraction by which the food bolus is carried down the oesophagus or any other segment of the alimentary canal.

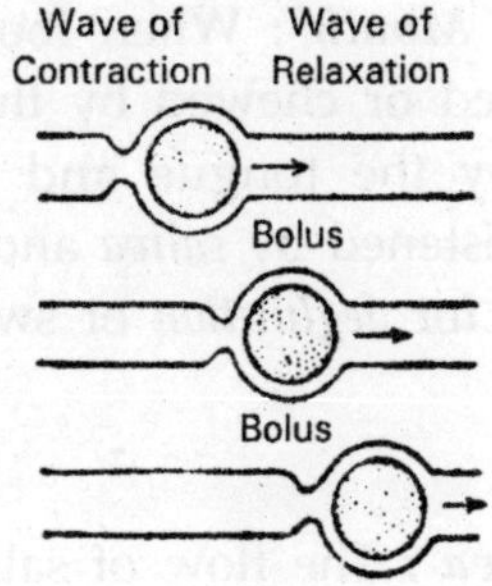

Peristalsis

Peristalsis may be defined as a wave of muscular contraction preceeded by a wave of relaxation which causes the contents of a hollow tube (gastro-intestinal tract) to be passed onwards. The circular muscles of the digestive tube immediately behind the bolus contract and those directly in front of it relax. This results in the bolus being forced into the relaxed portion. The contraction of muscles follows closely behind the bolus and further relaxation occurs in front of *L* ; thus the bolus of food passes steadily forwards.

Chemical Digestion : Chemical digestion is effected by the chemical substances, *enzymes* present in various digestive juices with which food comes in contact at different levels of alimentary tract. These enzymes catalyze the hydrolysis of native *proteins* to amino acids : of *starches* to monosaccharides ; and of *fats* to monoacylglycerols, glycerol and fatty acids. In the course of these digestive reactions, the *minerals* and *vitamins* of the food-stuffs are also made more assimilable.

The digestive juices, secreted in the various parts of the alimentary tract, are as follows :

Saliva in the mouth.

Gastric juice in the stomach.

Bile in the duodenum.

Pancreatic juice in the duodenum.

Intestinal juice (Succus entericus) in the small intestine.

Digestion in the Mouth : When food is taken into the mouth it is masticated or chewed by the teeth and moved round the mouth by the tongue and by the muscles of mastication. It is moistened by *saliva* and formed into a soft mass or bolus ready for *deglutition* or swallowing.

Saliva

Secretion of Saliva : The flow of saliva is controlled by sympathetic and parasympathetic nerve supply. The autonomic control of salivation occurs in two ways :

(i) *Unconditioned reflex* response to the presence of an object, such as food, in the mouth. This response may take place immediately after birth.

(ii) *Conditioned reflex* response is something which has been learned from previous experience. The sight, smell, and even thought of appetising food results in salivation sometimes called 'mouth watering'. This type of salivation occurs on the anticipation of food.

Composition of Saliva : Saliva is secreted into the mouth by 3 pairs of salivary glands ; parotids, submandibular and sublingual in *rabbit* ; parotids, submaxillary and sublingual in man. It consists of :

Water (99%)

Inorganic salts (0.2%) ; NaCl. KCl. Na_2HPO_4. $CaCO_3$.

$Ca(PO_4)_2$, KCNS.

Mucous (a glycoprotein) added by the glands in the mouth.

Enzymes; *ptyalin* or salivary a-amylase a bacteriolytic enzyme *lysozyme* and *lingual lipase.*

Functions of Saliva

(1) *Digestion :* Saliva contains a starch-splitting enzyme, salivary a amylase (ptyalin) that acts on cooked starches (polysaccharide) changing them into oligosaccharides : the disaccharide *maltose* the trisaccharide maltotriose and α-limit *dextrins*, branched polymers containing an average of about 8 glucose molecules.

Starch + Ptyaline $\longrightarrow$ Maltose + Maltotriose

(Polysaccharide) + α-limit dextrins.

Although saliva is capable of bringing about the hydrolysis of starch to maltose, this is of little significance in the body because of the short time it can act on the food. The pH of saliva is about 6.7 (slightly acidic).

(2) *Lubrication of Food :* Saliva moistens and lubricates the food; helping the formation of food masses suitable for swallowing.

(3) *Protection of Mouth Cavity :* It protects the delicate buccal mucous membrane by moisture the mouth and by diluting acids and other irritants.

(4) *Speech and Cleaning :* The mouth is kept constantly moist by the saliva which facilitates speech and cleaning of the buccal cavity by movements of the tongue.

(5) *Taste :* The taste buds are stimulated by particles present in the food which are dissolved in water. Dry foods stimulate the sense of taste only after thorough mixing with saliva.

(6) *Anti-bacterial Action :* Saliva contains as antibacterial enzyme 'Lysozyme' which dissolves the cell wall of many bacteria and finally kills them. This phenomenon justifies the common practice of sucking cut fingers.

Lingual lipase, secreted by glands on the tongue acts on triglycerides to some extent:

Triglycerides + Lingual lipase ⟶ Fatty acids.

+ 1, 2-diocylglycerols

In humans, about 1500 ml of saliva is secreted per day. Salivary secretion is easily conditioned, as shown in Favlov's experiments. In humans, the right, smell and even thought of food causes salivary secretion ("makes the mouth water").

Deglutition or Swallowing **:** Swallowing is a reflex response that is triggered by afferent impulses in the trigeminal, glassopharyngceal and vagus nerves. Swallowing of food occurs in three stages after mastication is complete and the bolus has been formed. The first two stages of swallowing are deliberate and voluntary. Subsequently, the individual has no further control and it becomes involuntary (a reflex action). The three stages as follows :

(i) The food bolus is pushed backwards into the pharynx by the upward movement of the tongue. The soft palate rises and shuts off the nasopharynx. At the same time the larynx is raised and its opening is occluded by the overhanging epiglottis.

(ii) The bolus is grasped into the pharynx by the contraction of the constrictor muscles and forced into the oesophagus.

(iii) The bolus of food is carried down the oesophagus by involuntary peristalis, and finally reaches the stomach. Inhibition of respiration and closure of glottis are part of the reflex response.

Digestion in the Stomach : Peristaltic action in the stomach consists of a *churning* movement which is brought about by contraction of the three layers of muscle fibres. This churning movement further causes mechanical breakdown of the food, mixing of the food with gastric juice and its onward movement into the duodenum.

Gastric Juice : There is always a small quantity of gastric juice present in the stomach, even when it contains no food. This is known as *fasting juice*. There are two phases of secretion of gastric juice:

(i) *Cephalic Phase :* The flow of juice occurs before food reaches the stomach and is due to reflex stimulation of the vagus nerves following the sight, smell or taste of food.

(ii) *Gastric Phase :* When stimulated by the presence of food (mainly protein), the gastric mucosa produced a hormone called gastrin which passes directly into the circulating blood, "is hormone stimulates the glands in the stomach wall to produce gastric juice.

In addition, alcohol and caffeine (present in tea, coffee and cold drinks) are potent stimuli for gastric release and thus acid secretion. A cocktail before dinner and a bowl of meat soup *i.e.* protein broth, before the main course both stimulate add secretion and prepare the stomach for the main meal. Besides these chemical stimuli, gastrin is also released in response to stimulation of parasympathetic fibres in the vagus nerve to the stomach.

Composition and Functions of Gastric Juice : In the mucosa of the stomach wall, 2 types of secretory glands are found ; those exhibiting a single layer of secretory cells (the chief cells), and those with cells arranged in layers (the parietal cells), which secrete directly into the gastric glands. The mixed secretion is known as gastric juice. It is normally a clear, pale yellow fluid of high acidity. 0.2—0.5% HCl, with a pH of about 1.0. The cells of the gastric glands secrete about 2500 of gastric juice daily. The gastric juice consists of:

Water
Hydrochloric acid
Enzymes ; pepsinogen, rennin and gastric lipase
Mucous
Inorganic salts
Intrinsic factor.

Water : The gastric juice is 97—99% water. Because of its watery consistency, it further liquefies the food swallowed.

Hydrochloric Acid : The parietal cells are the sole source of gastric hydrochloric acid. The functions of HCl are as follows:

(1) It acidifies the food and stops the action of ptyalin.

(2) Inactive pepsinogen is converted to the active enzyme pepsin by HCl.

$$\underset{\text{(Inactive)}}{\text{Pepsinogen}} \xrightarrow{\text{HCl}} \underset{\text{(Active)}}{\text{Pepsin}}$$

(3) The acid kills bacteria ingested with the food, thereby preventing their entry into the intestine.

Enzymes

Pepsin : The chief digestive function of the stomach is the parietal digestion of protein. Gastric pepsin is produced in the chief cells as the inactive zymogen, *pepsinogen,* which is activated to *pepsin* by the action of HCl and autocatalytically, by itself, *i.e.,* a small amount of pepsin can cause the activation of the remaining pepsinogen.

$$\text{Pepsinogen} \xrightarrow{H^+} \text{Pepsin}$$

$$\text{More Pepsinogen} \xrightarrow[\text{Pepsin itself}]{\text{Autocatalysis by}} \text{Pepsin}$$

The enzyme pepsin transforms native protein into proteoses and peptones which are still reasonably large protein derivatives.

(i) Pepsin + Proteins ⟶ Proteoses and Peptones.

(ii) Pepsin + Caseinogen (a phosphoprotein)

[Soluble Milk Protein]

$$\xrightarrow{\quad} \underset{\text{(Soluble)}}{\text{Casein}} \xrightarrow[\text{(Curdling)}]{\substack{\text{[Soluble Milk Protein]} \\ Ca^{++}}} \text{Ca Paracaseinate (Insoluble)}$$

$$\xrightarrow{\text{Pepsin}} \text{Proteoses and peptones}$$

Rennin (Chymosin, Rennet) : The enzyme causes the coagulation of milk. This is important in the digestive processes of calf because it prevents the rapid passage of milk from the stomach. In the presence of calcium, rennin changes irreversibly the casein of milk to a paracasein which is then acted on by pepsin.

Soluble milk protein caseinogen + Rennin—Insoluble Casein

$\xrightarrow{\text{Pepsin}}$ Proteoses and Peptones

Renin is said to be absent in the human gastric juice.

Mucous : It is a glycoprotein which helps to neutralize the acid in the stomach. Therefore, it reduces his gastric acidity and prevents injury to the gastric mucosa by forming a coating on the mucous membrane. The mucous also acts as a lubricant.

Inorganic Salts : These include NaCl, KCl, $CaCl_2$, $Ca(PO_4)_2$. $Mg(PO_4)_2$ and $MgHCO_3$ etc.

Intrinsic factor : Gastric juice contains the intrinsic factor (of Castle) which is necessary for the absorption of erythrocyte-maturing factor vitamin B_{12} (Cynacobalamin)'. The latter is sometimes called the Extrinsic Factor. Vitamin B_{12} is present in certain food stuffs ; is absorbed through the walls of the small intestine with the help of intrinsic factor and carried to the liver where it is stored. Vitamin B_{12} is essential for the proper development of the red blood cells in the bone marrow.

Regulation of Gastric Secretion : When the partially digested contents of the stomach reach the duodenum, particularly if they contain a considerable amount of fat, a hormone enterpogastrone is produced which slows down the secretion of gastric juice and reduces gastric motility.

Movements of the Stomach

The stomach acts as a temporary reservoir for food, thus allowing the digestive juices time to act on the different food substances. An ordinary meal takes about five hours to leave the stomach completely. During this period, the muscles of the stomach chum the food and mix it with water and gastric juice by waves of peristalsis passing from the upper part of the stomach towards the pylorus. The food which leaves the stomach to enter the duodenum is in a semiliquid state and this partially digested food material is called *chyme*. It passes into the duodenum in small jets when the pyloric sphincter relaxes and the muscular walls of the stomach contract.

Measures against Autodigestion of Stomach : Considering the high concentration of acid and proteolytic enzymes secreted by the stomach, it is natural to wonder why the stomach does not digest itself. Several factors protect the walls of stomach and duodenum.

Mucous Layer : The surface of the gastric mucosa is lined with cells which secrete a slightly alkaline mucous, which in humans forms a layer of 1 to 1.5 mm thick over the stomach surface. The protein content of mucous and its alkalinity tend to neutralize H^+ in the immediate area of the epithelial cell layer, thus forming a chemical barrier between the highly acid contents of the lumen and the cell surface. The mucous forms a flexible gel that coats the mucosa.

In addition, the cell membranes lining the stomach have a very low permeability to H^+, preventing their entry into the underlying mucosa.

Tight Junctions : The lateral surfaces of the epithelial cells near the lumen are joined together by tight junctions of cell membranes, so that there are no extracellular passage between the cells by which material could diffuse from the lumen into the mucosa.

Cell Replacement : The epithelial miscues cells lining the walls of the stomach are continually being shed and replaced through cell division so that the lining of the stomach is completely renewed every three days.

The above mentioned 3 factors contribute to maintaining a barrier between the contents of the lumen and the underlying tissues.

Hunger Contractions : Soon after the stomach is emptied, mild peristaltic contractions begin. They gradually increase in intensity over a period of hours. The more intense contractions can be felt as *hunger pangs.*

Intestinal Digestion : The stomach contents, or *chyme,* which are of a thick creamy consistency, are intermittently introduced during digestion into the duodenum through the pyloric valve. The pancreatic and bile ducts open the duodenum at a point very close to the Pylorus. The high alkaline content of biliary and pancreatic secretions neutralizes the acids of the chyme and changes the pH of this material to the alkaline side ; this shift of pH is necessary for the activity of the enzymes contained in the Pancreatic and intestinal juice.

The Bile : Bile is an alkaline viscous yellow to green bitter fluid (pH gold Human bile is yellowish green. In the carnivora it is golden yellow (due to the presence of more bilirubin), in herbivora the colour is green (due to more biliverdin) the bile is secreted continually by the liver at a rate of 0.5 to 1 litre per day. The gall bladder, a saccular organ attached to the hepatic duct, stroes a certain amount of the bile produced by the liver between meals. During digestion, the gall bladder contracts and supplies bile rapidly to the small intestine by way of the common bile duct. The pancreatic secretions mix with the bile, since they empty into the common duct shortly before its entry into the duodenum.

Secretion of Bile : Contraction of the gall bladder and relaxation of its sphincter are initiated by hormonal mechanism. The hormone Cholecystokinin (CCK) is secreted by the intestine in response to the presence of foods, mainly meats and fats. This hormone stimulates the gall bladder to undergo rhythmic contractions which result in an increase in the rate of flow of bile into the duodenum.

Composition and Functions of Bile : The gall bladder bile is more concentrated than the hepatic bile. In the gall bladder, water is absorbed and mucous is added, therefore, the bile gets concentrated and becomes a viscid fluid. The components of gall bladder bile are :

> Water, Mineral salts, Mucous, Bile salts, Bile pigments, Cholesterol and Lecithin.

Water : It constitutes about 86% of the bile.

Mineral Salts : These include Cl, CO_3 and PO_4 of Na, K, Ca and $NaHCO_3$. The latter neutralizes the acid chyme from the stomach.

Bile Salts : In the human bile there are two bile salts Potassium taurocholate (Bile Acids + Taurine), and Sodium, glycocholate (Bile Acids + Glycine) that are active in emulsifying fats in the duodenum. Emulsification is the breakdown of large fat globules into a suspension of very fine droplets 1 μ m in diameter. The fine droplets of fat, due to their innumerable number, provide the large surface area for the enzyme lipase to act upon. This quickens the process of digestion. The bile salts I have considerable ability to lower the surface tension of water. This enables them to emulsify fats in the intestine. The presence of bile in the small intestine is also necessary for the absorption of the fat-soluble vitamins A, D, E and K.

After transit through the small intestine, about 90% of the bile salts are actively absorbed in the ileum and carried to the liver by portal blood. From the liver, they are excreted in the bile back to the intestine. This process, which allows continued re-utilization of bilts salts, is termed the enterohepatic circulation' of the bile salts.

Bile Pigments : These are the waste products formed by the breakdown of haemoglobin of worn-out erythrocytes in the liver and are of no functional importance. Bile is their route of excretion. Bilirubin (golden-yellow) and biliverdin (green) are the most important bile pigments, Bilirubin is the chief pigment of human bile whereas biliverdin is the oxidation product of bilirubin.

Mucous : It acts as a buffer and a lubricant. *Cholesterol* and *Lecithin* (a phospholipid) are probably chiefly excretory products.

Besides the functions given above, bile is also an important vehicle of *excretion.* It removes many drugs, toxins and various inorganic substances such as copper, zinc and mercury. It colours and deodorizes the faeces.

Pancreatic Juice

Stimulation of Pancreatic Secretion : Like the stomach, the pancreas secretes its digestive juice almost entirely by means of hormonal stimulation. The hormones are secreted into the blood by the duodenum and upper jejunum as a result of stimulation by hydrochloric acid, fats, proteins, carbohydrates, and partially digested food stuffs. They are carried by the blood to the pancreas after absorption from the small intestine through the hepatic portal vein.

The active hormonal components formed by the duodenum (originally termed 'secretin' by Bayliss and Starling) have been separated into 2 separate factors :

(1) Secretin, which stimulates the production by the pancreas of a thin, watery fluid, high in bicarbonate but low in enzyme content :

(2) Pancreozymin, stimulating the production by the pancreas of a viscous fluid low in bicarbonate but high in enzyme content.

It was formerly thought that the cholecystokinin produced contractions of the gall bladder whereas a separate hormone called pancreozymin increased the secretion of pancreatic juice rich in enzymes. It has now become clear that a single hormone secreted by cells in the mucosa of the upper small intestine has both activities, and the hormone has therefore been named *cholecystokinin—pancreozymin.* It is also called *CCK — PZ* or most commonly, *CCK.*

Composition and Functions of Pancreatic Juice : Pancreatic juice is a nonviscid, alkaline fluid with a pH of 7.5 to 8.00. It consists of:

Water

Electrolytes : These are mainly Na^+, K^+, HCO_3^- and $C1^-$, Ca^{2+}, Zn^{2+}, HPO_4^{2-} and SO_4^{2-} are present in small amounts.

Acid chyme is rendered alkaline by the strong alkalinity o the pancreatic juice. This alteration is necessary for the effective action of the pancreatic enzymes.

Enzymes : These include trypsinogen, chymotrypsinogen amylase, lipase and peptidases.

Some of the pancreatic enzymes are secreted as inactive precursors (zymogens) such as trypsinogen and chymotrypsinogen, but are activated on contact with the intestinal mucosa. The activation of trypsinogen is attributed to *enterokinase,* which is produced by the intestinal glands. A small amount of active trypsin then autocatalytically activate additional trypsinogen and chymotrypsinogen.

$$\text{Trypsinogen} \xrightarrow[\text{intestinal juice}]{\text{Enterokinase of the}} \text{Trypsin}$$

Additional Trypsinogen; Chymotrypsinogen

$$\xrightarrow[\text{(Autocatalysis)}]{\text{Active Trypsin}} \text{Trypsin; Chymotrypsin}$$

Trypsin and Chymotrypsin : The protein-splitting action of pancreatic juice. (proteolytic action) is due to trypsin and chymotrypsin, which attack native protein, proteoses, and peptones from the stomach, converting them to tri- and dipeptides.

Trypsin, Chymotrypsin + Proteoses, Peptones ⟶ Small peptide chains

Chymotrypsin has more coagulative power for milk than trypsin, and as previously mentioned, it is activated not by enterokinase but by active trypsin.

Amylase : The starch-splitting action of pancreatic juice is due to a pancreatic enzyme *alpha-amylase.* It is similar in action to salivary amylase, hydrolyzing starch and glycogen to maltose, maltotriose and α-limit dextrins.

Amylase + Starch, Glycogen —— Maltose + Maltotriose

+ α-limit dextrins

Lipase : Fats are hydrolyzed by a pancreatic lipase to fatty acids, and glycerol.

Lipase + Emulsified fats → Fatty acids and 2-monoglycerides This is an important enzyme in digestion. Pancreatic lipase is specific for the hydrolysis of primary ester linkages such as occur in positions 1 and 3 of a triacylglycerol.

Carboxy Peptidase A : It acts on polypeptides clearing carboxy terminal amino acids that have aromatic or branched aliphatic side chains.

Carboxy Peptidase B : Acting on polypeptides, this enzyme cleaves carboxy terminal amino acids that have basic side chains.

Amino Peptidases : These act on polypeptides and cleave N-terminal amino acid from peptide.

Carboxy peptidases + Small peptide chains → smaller peptides.

Intestinal Juice

The intestinal juice is secreted by the specialized glands situated between the villi of the intestinal mucosa. It is alkaline in reaction (pH 8.0). This is the digestive juice which completes the digestion of carbohydrates, proteins and fats.

Stimulation and Intestinal Secretion : On entering the small intestine, chyme stimulates the mucous membrane to secrete the hormone enterocrinin which induces the flow of intestinal juice from intestinal glands.

Composition and Functions of Intestinal Juice.

The Intestinal juice consists of:

Water

Mineral Salts : Cl, HCO_3 and PO_4 of Na, K, Ca and Mg.

Mucous

Enzymes

The important enzymes and their functions are as follows:

(A) *Enterokinase* + Inactive Trypsinogen → Trypsin (active).

(B) Amino peptidedases + Smaller peptides → Dipeptides.

(C) Dipeptidases + Dipeptides → *Monopeptides (Amino Acids)*

(D) *Invertase (Sucrose)* + Sucrose → Glucose and Fructose.

(E) *Maltose or Glucoamylase* + Maltose, Maltotriose → Glucose

(F) α-limit dextrinase + α-limit dextrins → Glucose.

(G) *Lactose* + Lactose → Glucose and Galactose.

(H) *Lipase* + Remaining Emulsified fats → Fatty acids and Glycerol.

(I) *Phospholipase* + Phospholipids → Glycerol, Fatty acids Phosphoric acid.

(J) *Phosphatase* + Organic Phosphate → Free Phosphate.

(K) *Polynudeotidase* + Nucleic acid → Nucleotides.

(L) *Nucleosidases* + Purine or Pyrimidine Nucleosides → Purine or Pyrimidine bases + Pentose phosphate.

Major Products of Digestion

The final result of the action of the digestive enzymes already described is to reduce the food-stuffs of the diet to forms which can be absorbed and assimilated. These end products of digestion are, for carbohydrates, the monosaccharides (principally glucose) ; for *proteins*, the amino acids ; and for *triacyl-glycerol*, the fatty acids and glycerol.

Absorption from the Gastrointestinal Tract : Ingestion and digestion are the first two phases of the physiological processes occurring in the alimentary tract. The third phase is that of absorption.

Absorption from the Mouth : Normally, there is no absorption from the mouth, but a few drugs may be absorbed into the blood through the mucous membrane if allowed to dissolve under the tongue, e.g., *isoprenaline, glyceryl trinitrate.*

Absorption from the Stomach : In the stomach, absorption takes place to a limited degree. The only substances normally, absorbed from the stomach are some *water, glucose* and considerable amounts of *alcohol.* These substances are absorbed through the walls of the stomach into the venous circulation.

Although *iron* absorption takes place in the small intestine, it is dissolved out of foods most effectively in the stomach in the presence of HCl.

Absorption from the Small Intestine : The small intestine is the main absorptive organ. About 90% of the ingeted food-stuffs is absorbed in the course of passage through the small intestine. The surface area of the intestine through which absorption can take place is vastly increased by the circular folds *(plicae semilunares)* of the mucous membrane and by the large number of *villi.* The intestinal wall appears very much like a turkish towel. Surface area of the intestine is further increased by the microscopic folds, the *microvillu* protruding out from the surface of the intestinal epithelial cells.

There are 2 general pathways for the transport of materials absorbed by the intestine ; the veins of the hepatic portal system which lead directly to the liver; and the lymphatic vessels of the intestinal area, which eventually lead to the blood by way of the lymphatic system and the thoracic duct.

Absorption of Carbohydrates : The products of carbohydrate digestion are absorbed from the intestine into the blood of the portal venous system in the form of monosaccharides, chiefly the hexoses (glucose, fructose, mannose an galactose).

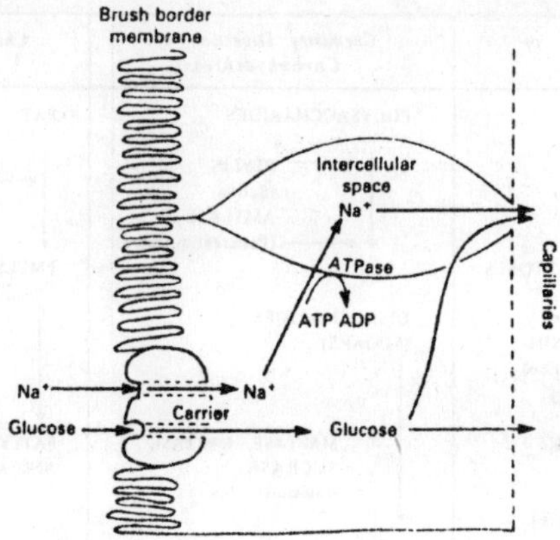

Mechanism for glucose transport across intestinal epithelium. Glucose transport into the intestinal cell is coupled to Na^+ transport utilizing a common carrier protein. Na^+ is then actively transported out of the cell and glucose diffuses into the capillaries.

Two mechanisms are responsible for absorption of monosaccharides : active transport against a concentration gradient and simple diffusion. To explain the active absorption of glucose, a mobile *carrier* has been postulated which binds both glucose and Na^+ at separate sites and which transports them both through the plasma membrane of the intestinal cell. It is envisaged that both the glucose and Na^+ are released into the eytosol, allowing the carrier to return for more "Cargo". Intracellular Na^+ is low, and Na^+ moves into the cell along its concentration gradient. Glucose moves with the sodium and is released in the cell.

The Na^+ is transported into the lateral intercellular spaces, and the glucose diffuses into the intestitium and thence to the capillaries. The energy for glucose transport is provided indirectly, by the active transport of Na^+ out of the cell. This maintains the concentration gradient across the luminal border of the cell, so that more Na^+ and consequently more glucose enter.

Chemical Digestion of Proteins	*Chemistry Digestion of Carbohydrates*	*Chemical Digestion of Fats*
PROTEIN FOOD	POLYSACCHARIDES	FAT
↓ ← PEPSIN (Gastric Juice)	↓ ← PTYLIN (Saliva) AMYLASE (Pancreatic Juice)	↓ ← BILE SALTS (Bile)
PROTEOSES AND PEPTONES		EMULSIFIED FATS
↓ TRYPSIN AND CHYMOTRYPSIN (Pancreatic Juice)	DISACCHARIDES (SUGARS)	↓ LIPASE (Pancreatic and Intestinal Juice)
TRI-AND DIPEPTIDES	↓ MALTASE, LACTASE SUCRASE (Intestinal Juice)	FATTY ACIDS AND GLYCEROL
↓ PEPTIDASES (Intestinal Juice)		
AMINO ACIDS (MONOPEPTIDES)	MONOSACCHARIDES (GLUCOSE, FRUCTOSE, GALACTOSE)	

Summary of Chemical Digestion of Food

The glucose mechanism also transports galactose.

Fructose is transported instead by facilitated diffusion. It utilizes a different carrier, and its absorption is independent of Na^+ or the transport of glucose and galactose. Some fructose is converted to glucose in the mucosal cells.

Pentoses are absorbed by simple diffusion.

Absorption or Amino acids and Protein : It is probable that under normal circumstances the dietary proteins are almost completely digested to their constituent amino acids and that these end products of protein digestion are then *actively transported* from the intestine into the portal blood.

Their exist several different carrier systems for transporting different classes of amino acids. Some of these required Na^+, just as in the case of carbohydrate transport.

Absorption of Fats : The dietary fat is digested, by the action of the pancreatic lipase. Fatty acids, monoglycerides and cholesterol in the intestine interact spontaneously with bile salts to form water soluble particles known as *micelles.* These cylindrical aggregates are 3—10 nm in diameter. Micellar formation solubilizes the lipids and provides a mechanism for their transport to mucosal cells of the ileum.

Monoglycerides, cholesterol, and fatty acids from the micelles enter the mucosal cells by passive diffusion. The subsequent fate of the fatty acids depends on their size :

(a) Fatty acids containing less than 10—12 carbon atoms pass from the mucosal cells directly into the portal blood where they are transported as free fatty acids.

(b) The fatty acids containing more than 10—12 carbon atoms are reesterified to triglycerides in the mucosal cells. The triglycerides are then coated with a layer of protein, cholesterol and phospholipid to form small lipid droplets about 0.5 μ m in diameter, known as *chylomicrons.* The latter are extruded by xocytosis from the basal or lateral aspects of the cell and passi nto the *lacteals* (lymph vessels) of the intestinal villi. By the lacteals, the fat is carried to the *cisterna chyli* (meaning the receiver of the chyle') and then by the thoracic (lymph) duct to the left branchiocephalic vein, where it enters the blood.

The lymph reaching the thoracic duct from the intestines contains an excess of fat giving it a milky appearance. It is called *chyle.*

In this way, fatty acids and glycerol are eventually brought into the blood stream and so, by a circuitous route, to the liver. In the liver, they are reorganized and recombined to form human fat.

In mucosal cells, most of the triglyceride is formed by the acylation of the absorbed 2-monoglycerides. However, some of the triglyceride is formed from glycerophosphate, which in turn is a product of glucose catabolism. Glycerophosphate is also converted into glycerophospholipids that participate in chylomicron formation.

Absorption of Vitamins : Waters and Vitamins as like members of B complex (except B_{12}) and vitamin C readily diffuse across the wails of the intestine into the blood. To move vitamin B_{12} across the wall of the ileum, a special system is required.

In the stomach, the vitamin combines with a special protein secreted by the gastric glands, known as the *intrinsic factor.* During the absorption process in the ileum, Vitamin B_{12} is released from the intrinsic factor and enters the blood.

The *fat-soluble vitamins,* vitamins A, D, E and K are dissolved in micells which enter the mucosal cells of the intestine by simple diffusion. The absorption of these fat-soluble vitamins is markedly decreased in the absence of bile.

Functions of the Large Intestine

(1) *Secretion :* The large intestine secretes mucine which lubricates the faeces and facilitates their passage through the rectum and anus.

(2) *Absorption :* As the food residues pass through the large intestine, water is absorbed by the walls of the colon

into the blood until the familiar semi-solid consistency of faeces is achieved. The absorption of water from the large intestine helps maintain the body water. Some drugs and mineral salts may also be absorbed into the blood from the large intestine but only very slowly.

(3) *Excretion :* Excess of calcium, iron and drugs of the heavy metal type such as bismuth are excreted by the large intestine.

Bacterial Decomposition of Cellulose

Defaecation : At fairly long intervals, a wave of strong pristasis sweeps along the transverse colon forcing its contents into the descending and pelvic colons. This is known as *mass movement* which is often precipitated by the entry of food into the stomach and is known as the *gastro-colic reflex*. When a mass movement forces the contents of the pelvic colon into the rectum, the nerve endings in the walls of the rectum are stimulated.

The act of defaecation, while reflex in the infant, in the adult is under the control of the will. The following actions occur during defaecation.

1. The sphincter muscle of the anus relaxes.
2. The muscular walls of the rectum contract.
3. The muscles of the floor of the pelvis contract.
4. The pressure within the abdomen is raised :
   (a) by holding the breath and contracting the diaphragm;
   (b) by contracting the muscles of the abdominal wall. The defaecation is carried out in response to the desire in children and adults, to empty the bowel production by distension of the rectum with faeces.

Constituent of Faeces : The faeces, consist of a semi-solid, paste-like mass coloured brown by *stercobilin,* a pigment derived from the bilirubin and biliverdin of the bile. It consists of:

Water (65—70% of the total bulk)

Under composed cellulose and other indigested fibre.

Protein residue (skatole, histidine, indole and tryptophan)

Dead and live micro-organisms.

Epithelial cells from the walls of the tract

Some fatty acids

Mucous secreted by the lining mucosa of the large intestine.

5

The Enzymes

Definition and History

Enzymes are protein catalysts for biochemical reactions in living cells. The term *enzyme,* derived from Greek means "in yeast" because the yeast cells were the first to reveal enzyme activity in living organisms. It was first introduced by W. Kuhne in 1878. Berzelius ; who was one of the first to define and recognize the nature of catalysts, proposed in 1827 that "ferments" were catalysts produced by living cells. In 1926 J.B. Stunner isolated the enzymes *urease* as a crystalline protein for the first time. He was awarded Nobel Prize in 1946 for this work. Since that time, several hundred enzymes have been obtained in highly purified form and more than 150 of these in the crystalline state. The study of enzymes, nowadays, is dealt with under a separate branch of Biochemistry, known as the *enzymology*.

Enzymic reactions were used by man long before written history. The discovery of fermentation to produce wines was attributed by the Greeks to Bacchus. The making of cheese, the leavening of bread, and the manufacture to vinegar are enzymic processes that stem from the ancient times. These practical activities have occupied an important place in the history of enzymology.

The breweries and their research laboratories have provided much information concerning the processes by which living cells utilize sugar because the fundamental reactions of fermentation in a yeast culture are much the same as in the tissues of mammals. Indeed, the name enzyme, coined by Kuhne means "in yeast", but the word is now used to denote a biological catalyst, regardless of origin.

A substantial part of the study of living cells is today devoted to enzymes inasmuch as all physiological functions *e.g.* muscular contraction, nerve conduction, excretion etc., as well as life itself are intimately linked to the activity of enzymes.

Nomenclature : Enzymes are named in a variety of ways:

(1) A customary practice is to add the suffix *-ase* to the name of the substrate, *i,e.*, the substance on which the enzyme acts upon. For example, the enzyme that attacks urea by *urease*, arginine is acted upon by *arginase*, *tyrosine* by *tyrosinase*, uric acid by *uricase*, amylum (starch) by *amylase* etc.

(2) Enzymes may also be named by groups that catalyze similar chemical reactions such as *dehydrogenases*, *oxidases*, *proteinases*, *Upases*, *glycosidases*, *decarboxylases etc.*

(3) The suffix *-lytic* is used to denote enzyme activity on class of substrates such as *proteolytic* for protein-splitting, *lipolytic* for the (lipos) — splitting, and *sucrolytic* for enzymes acting upon carbohydrates.

(4) A few enzymes retain their old traditional nomenclature, and we find such names as *ptyalin*, *pepsin*, *rennin*, *trypsin* etc.

(5) Some proteinases of plants and microorganisms have been named from the species of origin *e.g. pepain* from papaya, *Jicin* from ficus,*subtilisin* from Bacillus *substilis* etc.

Classification : According to International Union of Biochemistry (IUB), the present system of classification of enzymes is based on their reaction specificity. Six classes have been recognized :

1. Oxidoreductases (Catalyze oxidation-reduction reactions)

   This class includes enzymes which are concerned with biological oxidation and reduction, and therefore, with respiration and fermentation processes. The important subclasses are :

   (i) Dehydrogenases, that catalyze reactions in which the electron transfer is accompanied by the transfer of hydrogen atoms *e.g., alcohol dehydrogenase* and *glutamic dehydrogenase* of animal liver.

   (ii) Oxidases, in which molecular oxygen is one of the reactants *e.g., cytochrome oxidase.*

   (iii) Peroxidases, which use H_2O_2 as the oxidant.

   (iv) Oxygenases, which introduce molecular oxygen in place of a double bond in the substrate.

2. Hydrolases (catalyze hydrolytic reactions). These fall into 3 categories :

   (A) *Proteases (Proteolytic enzymes).* These are enzymes that attack the peptide bonds of proteins and peptides. It is customary to distinguish between the proteinase (endopeptidases) and the peptidases (exopeptidases).

   (a) *Peptidases (Exopeptidases)* act on peptide bonds adjacent to a free amino or carboxyl group. Among the principal types are the following :

(i) *Carboxypeptidases* require a free α -carboxyl group in the substrate and split the peptide bond adjacent to this group, liberating a free amino acid.

(ii) *Aminopeptidases* act on the peptide bond adjacent to the free amino group of the simple peptides.

(iii) *Dipeptidases* specifically act on certain dipeptides. An example is *glycylglycine dipeptidase* which requires CO^{2+} or Mn^{2+} for its action.

(b) *Proteinases (Endopeptidases)* act on the interior peptide bonds of proteins; they can, however, also split peptide bonds in suitable simple peptides and their derivatives. Examples are *pepsin, rennin, trypsin, chymotrypsin* and *plasmin* from animals.

Catnepsins are intracellular proteinases found in most animal tissues. The richest sources are liver, kidney and spleen.

Plant Proteinases : *Papain* is obtained from the unripe fruit of the papaya. Similar enzymes are *bromelin,* found in pineapples and *Jicin* in the milky sap of the fig tree.

(B) *Esterases :* These enzymes catalyze hydrolysis of ester linkages. Classification depends on both the type of acid and the type of alcohol constituting the ester.

(a) *Simple esterases* such as *esterase* which catalyzes reversibly the scission and synthesis of esters of lower alcohols and fatty acids.

(b) *The true Upases* hydrolyze fats into long-chain fatty acids and glycerol. Examples are *pancreatic Upase* and plant *Upases.*

(c) *Phosphatases* hydrolyze esters of phosphoric acid.

(d) *Pyrophosphatases* hydrolyze pyrophosphate linkages.

(e) *Nucleases* cause hydrolysis of nucleic acids, liberating aligo- or mononucleoitides. These enzymes are *phospho-diesterases.*

(C) *Carbohydrases* : These enzymes hydrolyze the glycosidic linkages of simple glycosides, oligosaccharides, and polysaccharides.

(a) *Glycosidases* hydrolyze simple glycosides and oligosaccharides. An example is yeast *invsrtase,* which hydrolyzes sucrose to glucose and fructose.

(b) *Polysaccharidases* act on complex polysaccharides.

β-amy lases hydrolyze starch and glycogen to maltose and to residual polysaccharides. The polysaccharides of wheat, barley, soyabeans and other plants are of this type.

α-amylases can hydrolyze glycogen and starch and the residual polysaccharides of starch (amylodextrins) to give glucose, maltose, and product that no longer give a colour with iodine. Animal amylase of this type have been obtained in crystalline form from pancreas and saliva. These are also found in blood and urine.

Transferases (Catalyze group transfer reactions) : These enzymes catalyze the transfer of a group from one substance to another. The groups may be alkyl, glycosyl, acyl, amino, aldehyde, sulphur or phosphorus.

(i) Acyltransfereases, *e.g. choline acyltransferase.*

(ii) Glycosyltransferases, *e.g., phosphorylase.*

(iii) Aminotransferases or Transaminases, *e.g. glytamic-aspartic aminotransferase.*

(iv) *Kinases.* Enzymes catalyzing transfer of a phosphate

group, specifically from the ATP to particular substrates, *e.g., hexokinase.*

Lyases : (Catalyze removal of groups from substrates by mechanisms other than hydrolysis, leaving double bonds).

$$\begin{array}{ccc} X & & Y \\ | & & | \\ C - C & = X - Y + & C = C \end{array}$$

These enzymes act on C—C, C—O, C—N, C—S and C—halide bonds. The important ones are as under :

(i) *Hydrases (Carbon-oxygen lyases)* : These enzymes catalyze addition to or removal of water from their specific substrates. For examples, *fumarase* catalyzes the intercon-version of malic and fumaric acids ;

$$HOOC—CH_2—CHOH—COOH = HOOC—CH — CH—COOH + H_2O$$

Malic acid *Fumaric acid*

(ii) Aldehyde-Lyases, *e.g., Aldolase.*

(iii) *Decarboxylases* : These enzymes remove CO_2 from carboxylic acids. *Keto add decarboxylases* are important in the liberation of CO_2. An example is the catalyzed decarboxylation of pyruvic acid to acetaldehyde and CO_2.

$$CH_3COCOOH \xrightarrow{\text{Decarbaxylase}} CH_3CHO + CO_2$$

Isomerases (Catalyze isomeration reactions) : These enzymes catalyze intramolecular rearrangements, *e.g.*, the interconversion of aldose and ketose sugars. For example, *phosphohexose isomerase* catalyzes the following interconversion :

$$\text{Glucose 6-Phosphate} \rightleftharpoons \text{Frunctose 6-phosphate}$$

In this group of enzymes are also included the *epimerases, e.g., uridine diphosphate galactose 4-epimerase,* which catalyzes the following reaction :

Uridine diphosphate galactose ⇌ Uridine diphosphate glucose.

Uridine diphosphate glucose plays an important role in several aspects of carbohydrate metabolism.

Other examples of isomerases are *alanine recemase* and *retinene isomerase.*

Ligases or Synthetases : (Ligare = "to bind". Catalyze synthesis by condensation of two groups requiring ATP or a similar triphosphate).

These enzymes catalyze reactions forming C—O, C—S, C—N and C—C bonds. Some sub-classes are :

(i) Enzymes, catalyzing formation of C—S bonds, *e.g. succinic thiokinase.*

(ii) Enzymes, catalyzing formation of C—N bonds, *e.g., glutamine synthetase.*

(iii) Enzymes, catalyzing formation of C—C bonds, *e.g., acetyl COA carboxylase.*

Chemical Nature of Enzymes : Enzymes are the largest and most specialized class of protein molecules. They are of two types : simple and holoenzymes.

1. *Simple Enzymes :* Some enzymes are simple proteins, *i. e.*, on hydrolysis, they yield amino acids only. Digestive enzymes such as *pepsin, trypsin,* and *chymotrypsin* are of this nature.
2. *Conjugated Enzymes :* Many enzymes possess chemical groups that are non-amino acid in nature. These conjugated proteins are called *holoenzymes. A* holoenzyme may be dissociated into a protein component, termed the *apoenzyme* and a non-protein moeity, the *cofactor.* Cofactors may be divided into 3 groups which include : (a) prosthetic groups, (b) coenzymes, and (c) metal activators.

Conjugated protein enzyme $\rightleftharpoons$ Apoenzyme (Protein part)

or Holoenzyme

\+ Non-protein cofactor (Prosthetic group/Coenzyme/Metal activator)

(a) *Prosthetic Group* : *A* prosthetic group is firmly bound to the enzyme protein. Thus, for example, the *porphyrin* part of the enzyme. Haemoprotein peroxidase and FAD in succinic dehydrogenase are prosthetic groups that are firmly associated With their protein counter. Combination of an apoenzyme parts, and a co-factor with the substrate.

(b) *Coenzyme : A* coenzyme is a small, heat-stable, dialyzable organic molecule which readily dissociates off an enzyme protein. Thus, NAD, *NADP, Thiamine pyrophosphate* and *Tetrahydro folic acid* are examples of coenzymes.

(c) *Metal Activator* : An enzyme may contain only amino acids and a metal. For example, here are enzymes that are copper proteins; *ascorbic acid oxidase* is one of them. In this enzyme Cu is tightly bound and is not separated readily from the protein apoenzyme. Many other enzyme require metal ions for their activation. The ions of Ca, Co, Cu, Mg, Mn, Mo, Na, K and Zn are known to participate in enzymic reactions. In some cases these *activators* function in combination with the protein, in others the metal ion forms a compounds with a substrate.

Endo and Exoenzymes

Enzymes which act only within the cells are called *endoenzymes,* hence they are metabolic enzymes *e.g., cytochrome oxidase.* On the contrary, certain enzymes are liberated by living cells and catalyze vital reactions in the cell's environment.

These are called *exoenzymes e.g.*, the digestive enzymes : *amylase, lipase, proteases* etc.

General Properties of Enzymes

(1) *Remain Unaltered in the End :* One of the primary characteristics of enzymes is their emergence from a reaction or set of reactions in an *unaltered* state. This enzyme may now enter into another reaction with another substrate of the same type.

(2) *Required in Small Quantities :* Enzymes are active in small quantities. Since the enzyme is reused, only a small quantity of an individual enzyme is required by biological systems. It has been estimated that a single enzyme can act upon 500,000 substrate molecules per minute. This value is referred to as the *turnover number.*

(3) *Protein Nature :* The third general property of enzymes is their protein nature. The protein structure provides for weak associations due to side groups of the amino acids within it. The enzyme—substrate complex involves the association of the enzyme and substrate by weak associations rather than covalent bondings. Enzymes exhibit all typical properties of proteins *viz*.. High molecular weight, colloidal behaviour, slow diffusion, inability to pass through most living membranes, and movement in response to an electric current.

(4) *Accelerate the Rate of Reaction : An enzyme changes only the rate of the reaction,* not the direction of the equilibrium. A reaction will proceed at a faster rate in the presence of an enzyme, but the equilibrium between the substrase and the product will remain constant with or without the intervention of the enzyme.

(5) *Reversibility of Enzyme Action :* Certain enzymes exhibit reversibility of their action. This property is very helpful

in metabolism. For example, *succinic dehydrogenase* catalyzes reversibly the dehydrogenation of succinic acid (in the presence of a suitable hydrogen acceptor A) of hydrogenation of fumaric acid.

(6) *Enzyme Specificity* : The specificity of enzymes is one of their most fundamental and important properties. By contrast to non-protein catalysts (H^+, OH^- or metal ions), enzymes catalyze only one specific reaction or act upon only one kind of substrate. The specificity may be of any kind, *e.g.*, reaction specificity, substrate specificity, group specificity or optical specificity.`

(i) *Reaction Specificity* : Most enzymes can catalyze the same type of reaction (phosphate transfer, oxidation-reduction etc.) with several structurally related substrates. For example, some esterases can act upon the esters different fatty acids with a variety of alcohols. Nevertheless, the esterases are specific in their esterase actions, they do not catalyze other hydrolytic reactions, nor do they function as oxidises, decarboxylases etc. Specificity is evident in the type of reaction that is catalyzed.

(ii) *Substrate Specificity* : A very important feature of enzyme activity is that it is *substrate specific i. e.*, a particular enzyme will act only on a certain substrate. For example, *urease* is a specific enzyme, it acts on urea only but it would not exert any influence on the catabolism of protein or carbohydrate.

(iii) *Group Specificity* : A particular enzyme acts only on particular chemical groupings *e.g. glycosidase* on glycosides, *alcohol dehydrogenase* on alcohols, *pepsin* and *trypsin* on peptide bonds and esterases on ester linkages. *Chymotrypsin* preferentially hydrolyzes peptide bonds in which the carboxyl group is contributed by the aromatic amino acids phenylalanine, tyrosine, or typtophan. *Carboxypeptidases* and *aminopepti- doses* split of amino acids one at a time from the carboxyl or amino terminal end of polypeptide chains, respectively.

(vi) *Optical Specificity (Stereospecificity)* : With the exception of *epimerases* which interconvert optical isomers, *emzyme generally show absolute optical specificity for at least a portion of a substrate molecule.*

Thus maltase catalyzes the hydrolysis of α - but not β -glycosides, while enzymes of the Embden-Meyerhof and direct oxidative pathways catalyze the inter-conversion of D- but not L-phosphosugars. With a few exception, such as the D-amino acid oxidase of kidney, the vast majority of mammalian enzymes act on the L-isomers of amino acids. An example of stereospecificity among enzymes is the conversion of pyruvic acid to lactic acid by reduction. This process can be accomplished by two different enzymes, each producing but one of the optical isomers :

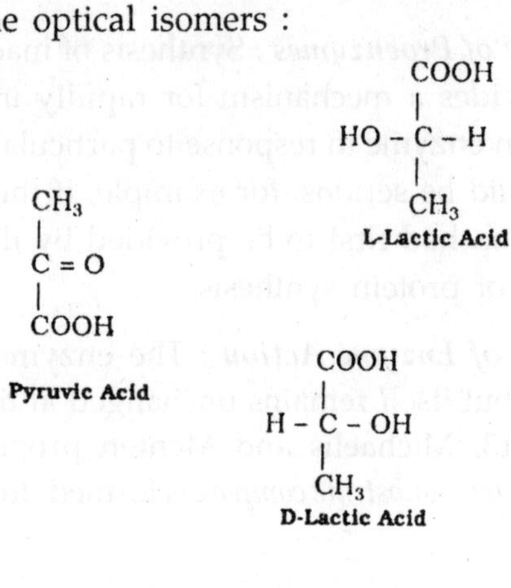

Proenzymes

Some enzymes are produced in a catalytically inactive or pro-enzyme form which must undergo limited proteolysis, to become catalytically active. This phenomenon is best illustrated by certain digestive enzymes, as well as by enzymes of blood coagulation and of blood clot dissolution.

Conversion of the proenzyme to the active enzyme is catalyzed either by proteolytic enzymes or by hydrogen ions:

$$\text{Pepsinogen} \xrightarrow{H^+ \text{ or Pepsin}} \text{Pepsin}$$

$$\text{Tripsinogen} \xrightarrow{\text{Trypsin or Enterokinase}} \text{Trypsin}$$

$$\text{Chymotrypsinogen} \xrightarrow{\text{Trypsin}} \text{Chymotrypsin}$$

$$\text{Procarboxypeptidase} \xrightarrow{\text{Trypsin}} \text{Carboxypeptidase}$$

Since activation of proenzyme is catalyzed by the active form of the enzyme itself, the activation of pepsinogen and of trypsinogen proceeds with ever-increasing velocity and is said to be *autocatalytic*.

Conversion of fibrinogen to fibrin involves limited proteolysis catalyzed by thrombin. Under normal physiologic conditions, thrombin exists as the inactive precursor, prothrombin, and its activation requires a complex sequence of reactions.

Significance of Proenzymes : Synthesis of inactive enzyme precursors provides a mechanism for rapidly increasing the availability of an enzyme in response to particular physiologic demand. It would be serious, for example, if the enzymes of blood coagulation had first to be provided by the somewhat slower process of protein synthesis.

Mechanism of Enzyme Action : The enzyme promotes a given reaction, but itself remains unchanged at the end of the reaction. In 1913, Michaelis and Menten proposed that an intermediate *enzyme-substrate complex* is formed during enzymic activity. The following scheme may be written to illustrate concept:

$$\text{Enzyme (E) + Substrate (S)} \rightleftharpoons \text{Enzyme-Substrate Complex (ES)} \rightarrow \text{Enzymes + Products (P)}$$

The enzyme itself remains almost passive. It merely provides a "platform" *or template* on which certain molecules could react with each other. Such an enzyme-platform brings reacting molecules into contact much faster than chance collisions at that temperature. The result is that the reactions are accelerated.

Enzymes Reduce the Energy of Activation : The effect of enzymes is to lower the activation-energy requirements, thereby promoting appreciable reaction rates at lower temperatures than would be possible otherwise. *Energy of activation is that minimal amount of energy which is required of a molecule to take part in a reaction.* For example, decomposition of hydrogen peroxide without a catalyst has an energy activation of some 18,000 ca/mole. When the enzyme *catalase* is added, it is less than 2,000.

Enzymes Accelerate Reactions by Reducing the free Energy of Activation : According to this concept, reactants A and B, in order to react to form the product C, must pass through a transition state (A - B) in which the activated complex is formed and certain amount of activation energy (E) is required. When the proper enzyme is present, less energy is required for activation (E_a'). In other words, the combination of substrate with enzyme creates a new-reaction pathway that has a transition state of lower energy than in the absence of enzyme.

The Catalytic Site

The larger size of protein-enzymes compared to their substrates led biochemists in the beginning of the century to postulate that some restricted region of the enzyme was concerned with the process of catalysis. This region was termed as the *active site.* Now-a-days, we refer to the catalytic site, since it is now known that other sites are also "active" (*e.g.*, allosteric sites). Although enzymes differ widely in structure, specificity, and mode of catalysis, a number of generalizations concerning their catalytic sites can be stated as follows :

1. *The catalytic sites take up a relatively small portion of the total volume of an enzyme.* It is interesting to note that most of the amino acid residues in an enzyme are not in contact with the substrate.

2. *The Catalytic Site is a Three-dimensional Entity* : The catalytic site of an enzyme is not a point, a line, or even a plane. It consists of *contact* amino acid residues, which are fairly close to each other in the native structure of the enzyme because of the three-dimensional folding of the molecule, but may be actually far apart in the primary sequence. For example, in *lysozymes* the important groups in the catalytic site are contributed by residues numbered 35,52,62,63 and 101 in the linear sequence of 129 amino acids.

3. *Catalytic sites are clefts or crevices.* In all enzymes, substrate molecules are bound to a cleft or crevice from which water is largely excluded.

4. *Substrates are Bound to Enzymes by Relatively Weak Forces* : The binding of the substrate to the catalytic site involve forces of a non-covalent nature (ionic and hydrogen bonds, Vander Waals forces), which are of very short range.

***The Interaction of Substrates and Enzymes* :** The mechanism of enzyme action has been explained by two theories: *Lock and Key* theory of Emil Fischer and *Induced fit* theory of Koshland.

***Lock and Key Theory (Rigid Model of the Catalytic Site)* :** The original model of a catalytic site, proposed by Emil Fisher in 1890, visualized interaction between substrate and enzyme in terms of a "lock and key". Just as only particularly shaped keys fit into particularly shaped locks, similarly, only certain types of molecules will establish a close fit with a given type of enzyme protein. This concept was developed to explain the great specificity of enzymes. According to this concept, a structurally well defined catalytic site will accept only those substrate molecules which have a matching shape and will repell others that differ structurally. In other words, the catalytic site of the enzymes by itself is complementary in shape to that of the substrate.

Induced Fit Theory (Flexible Model of the Catalytic Site) **:** An essential feature of the "induced fit" model of Koshland is the flexibility of the region of catalytic site. In the Fischer model, the catalytic site is presumed to be pre-shaped to fit the substrate. In the induced fit model, the substrate induces a *conformational change* in the enzyme. According to this postulate, the catalytic sites of some enzymes are not rigid. In these enzymes, the shape of the catalytic site is modified by the binding of substrate. The catalytic site has a shape complementary to that of the substrate only after the substrate is bound. This process of dynamic recognition is called induced fit. It brings amino acid residues or other groups on the enzyme in the correct spatial orientation for substrate binding, catalysis or both. At the same time, other amino acid residues may become burried in the interior of the enzyme molecule.

Factors Affecting Enzyme Activity

(1) *Temperature* : Between a range of 0°C and 45°C, the activity of the enzymes in increased when the temperature is raised, as in most chemical reactions. It has been found that a rise of 10°C hastens the reaction 2 or 3 times. The increase is due to two factors : (i) the influence of heat on the chemical reaction itself and (ii) the increased enzyme activity.

The rate of enzyme catalyzed reactions do not, however, increase indefinitely as the temperature is increased. At some point, usually in the range between 45° to 60°C, thermal denaturation will destroy the catalytic function of the enzyme protein. As the enzyme is inactivated, the reaction which it catalyzes, slows down and ultimately stops. There is thus, an optimum temperature for each enzyme.

Most enzymes operate at their best in a temperature range of about 25° to 40°C (human body temperature is 37°C) however, certain enzymes are very resistant to high temperature. For example, crystalline trypsin is denatured reversibly even at 100°C and so is Taka Diastase.

(2) *Hydrogen Ion Concentration (pH)* : One of the most interesting environmental influences on enzymatic activity is the effect of pH. Each enzyme is catalytically active within a limited range of pH. Though each particular type of enzyme has its own specific optimum, most enzymes operate effectively in a pH range of about 5.0 to 9.0. For example, the optimal range for the activity of *malt amylase* is 5.2 ; for *salivary amylase,* between 6.7 and 6.8 ; for *trypsin,* between 8 and 11. However, a few enzymes *e.g. pepsin* are active at pH values between 1.5 and 2.5. In all these cases activity declines gradually on either side of the optimum. In addition to the purely, ionic effects, extremes of pH values can cause considerable denaturation and hence inactivation of the enzyme protein.

(3) *Enzyme Concentration :* The rate of a chemical reaction influenced by a particular enzyme, in most cases, increses proportionally with increasing concentration of the enzyme, ' provided that the substrate is present abundantly and is therefore not rate limiting.

(4) *Substrate Concentration* : At a constant concentration of enzyme, the reaction rate increases with increasing substrate concentration until a maximal velocity is reached. At a sufficiently high substrate concentration, the catalytic sites are filled and so the reaction rate reaches a maximum. Therefore, further increase in concentration of substrate has no effect on the rate of the reaction. In contrast, uncatalyzed reactions do not show this saturation effect.

(5) *Cofactors* : Some enzymes require small non-protein components called *cofactors* for their activity. For example, the *cytochromes* are conjugated proteins having tightly bound *prosthetic groups.* The cytochromes have a metalloporphyrin complex and are involved in electron-transfer reactions.

(6) *Chemical Substances* : It has been found that the activity of many hormones and certain drugs results from inhibition or exhancement of enzyme action.

Enzyme Kinetics

The kinetic characteristics of enzymes can best be illustrated by a graph (Fig.). Without having anything to react with, the

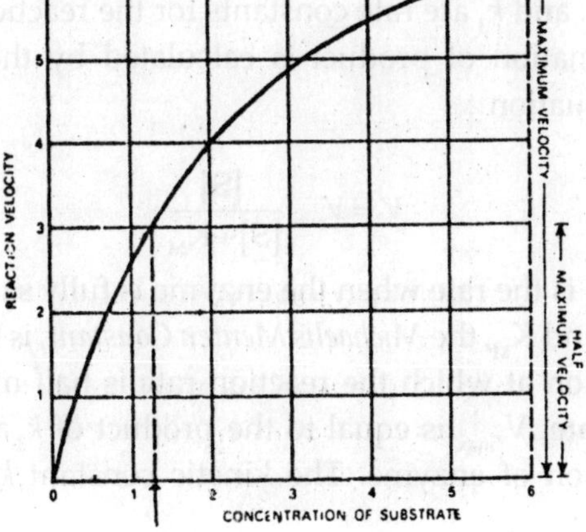

enzyme will not show any activity. Therefore, assuming a ready supply of enzyme, the apparent activity will increase with the availability of the substrate. However, as the substrate supply increases, a point will be reached when all available enzyme molecules will be fully employed ; this is the point of *maximum velocity* of reaction for a given enzyme concentration with a given substrate. Obviously, this point will vary according to the enzyme and the substrate, and is a measure of the detailed mechanism of enzyme action on the particular substrate. We can also note the halfway point to this maximum velocity and measure the amount of substrate necessary to reach it. The amount of substrate required for half-maximal velocity is called the *Michaelis-Menten Constant*. It gives some measure of the affinity the enzyme and the substrate have for one another.

Michaelis-Menten Model of Enzyme Kinetics : In 1913, Leonor Michaelis and Maud Menten proposed a simple model to account for the kinetic characteristics of many enzymes. In this model, the enzyme (E) combines with a substrate (S) to form an enzyme-substrate (ES) complex, which can proceed to form product (P) or dissociate into E and S.

$$E+S \underset{k_2}{\overset{k_1}{\rightleftharpoons}} ES \xrightarrow{k_3} E+P$$

where k_1, k_2 and k_3 are rate constants for the reactions. The rate (V) of formation of product is calculated by the Michaelis-Menten equation :

$$V = V_{\max} \frac{[S]}{[S]+K_M}$$

where V_{max} is the rate when the enzyme is fully saturated with substrate, and K_M, the *Michaelis Menten Constant*, is the substrate concentration at which the reaction rate is half maximal. The maximal rate, V_{max} is equal to the product of k_3 and the total concentration of enzyme. The kinetic constant k_3, called the turnover number, is the number of substrate molecules converted into product per unit time by a single catalytic site when the enzyme is fully saturated with substrate. Turnover number for most enzymes are between 1 and 10^4 per second.

Enzyme Inhibition : Enzymes can be inhibited by specific small molecules or ions. The inhibition of enzymes serves as a major control mechanism in biological systems. Certain enzyme inhibitors such as cyanide, carbon monoxide, oxalic acid etc, are *poisonous* for living organisms. Their toxicity is due to their ability to inhibit enzymic reactions. On the other hand, an inhibitor blocking a disease producing reaction represents a *medicinal drug*. It is thought that the action of sulphonamides in killing bacteria, or preventing their reproduction, may be due to a similar interference with enzyme system in the bacterial cell. Furthermore, enzyme inhibition can provide insight into the mechanism of enzyme action. Some of the strongest evidence for the localization of catalytic sites comes from studies with specific inhibitors of enzymes. By specific inhibitors are meant compounds that can combine with an enzyme in such a manner as to prevent the normal enzyme-substrate combination and the catalytic reaction.

Enzyme inhibition may be *reversible* or *irreversible.*

Reversible Inhibition : This type of enzyme inhibition is characterized by a rapid equilibrium of the inhibitor and enzyme. There are two major types of reversible inhibition : (a) Competitive and (b) Non-competitive.

(a) *Competitive or Surface Analog Inhibition :* Competitive inhibition involves a compound which resembles the substrate and binds to the catalytic site of the enzyme. The substrate is then prevented from binding to the same active site. The formation of an enzyme-inhibitor complex may be represented as

$$E + I \rightleftharpoons EI$$

where E is the enzyme, I the inhibitor, and EI the enzyme-inhibitor complex.

In competitive inhibition, the formation of EI is reversible and their is continuing competition between the substrate and the inhibitor for the same locus on the enzyme. This situation is, therefore, designated as "competitive inhibition". The actual rate of the catalyzed reaction is then strictly dependent on the relative concentrations of substrate and inhibitor. The inhibition can be reversed by increasing the substrate concentration so that the substrate molecules outnumber those of the inhibitor.

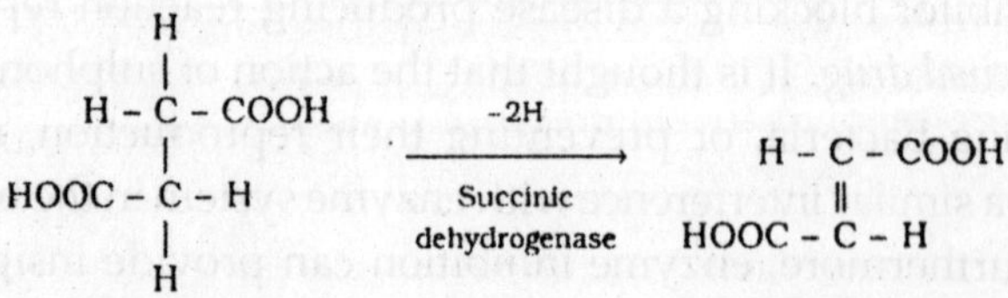

Succinic Acid   Fumaric Acid

A classic example of competitive inhibition is the action of malonic acid on succinic dehydrogenase. An enzyme that dehydrogenates acid.

Many compounds that are structurally similar to succinic acid but which are not dehydrogenated can combine with the enzyme and inhibit catalysis of the normal reaction by blocking the "active site" of the enzyme. The inhibition of succinic dehydrogenase by malonic acid, whose molecular structure is very similar to that of succinic acid, serves as an example of competitive inhibition :

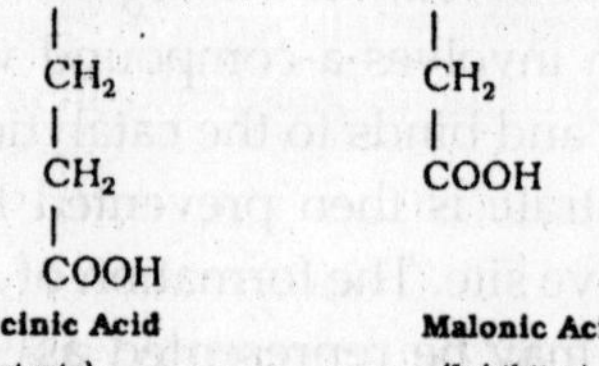
Succinic Acid (Substrate)   Malonic Acid (Inhibitor)

Enzyme = *Succinic dehydrogenase.*

In this case, both the substrate (succinic acid) and the inhibitor (malonic acid) will compete for the active (catalytic) site, and the enzyme activity will be reduced. Compounds like oxalic acid, glutaric acid and phenyl propoionic acid also inhibit succinic dehydrogenase. This inhibition can be reversed by increasing the substrate concentration, so that the substrate molecules outnumber those of inhibitor. One more example of competitive inhibition is shown below :

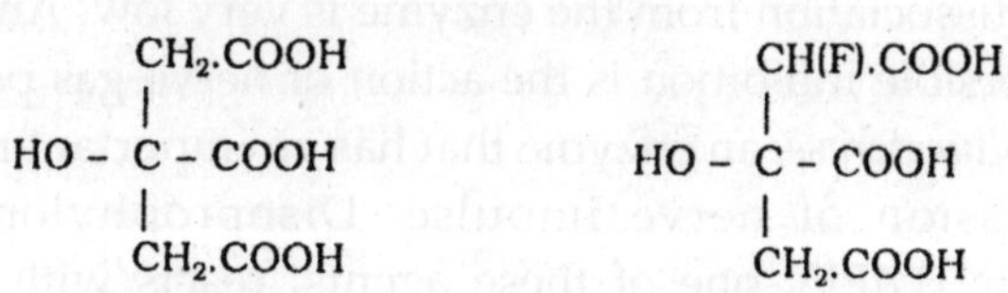

Citric Acid (Substrate) **Fluorocitric Acid** (Inhibitor)

A physiologically important example of competitive inhibition is found in the formation of 2,3-Diphosphoglycerate from 1, 3 Di-phosphoglycerate. *Diphosphoglycerate mutase,* the enzyme catalyzing this isomerization, is competitively inhibited by low levels of 2, 3-Diphosphoglycerate. In such a case the product of an enzymatic reaction has a structural resemblance to the substrate and, therefore, it serves as a competitive inhibitor.

Non-Competitive Inhibition : In this type, the Inhibitor and the substrate are not structurally related ; they can bind simultaneously to an enzyme molecule. This means that their binding sites do not overlap. Since these inhibitors bear no structural resemblance to the substrate, an increase in the substrate concentration generally is ineffective in relieving this inhibition.

A non-competitive inhibitor acts by decreasing the turnover number of an enzyme rather than by diminishing the proportion of enzyme molecules that have a bound substrate. In contrast to the competitive type, it may be assumed that the formation of EI in non-competitive inhibition occurs at a locus on the enzyme that is not attacked by the substrate. $E + I \rightleftharpoons EI$ and $ES + I \rightleftharpoons ESI$

where EI and ESI are inactive.

Reversible, non-competitive inhibition is, in any case, rare.

Irreversible Inhibition : In this type of inhibition, the inhibitor is covalently linked to the enzyme or bound so tightly that its dissociation from the enzyme is very low. An example of irreversible inhibition is the action of nerve gas poisons on *acetylcholinesterase*, an enzyme that has an important role in the transmission of nerve impulse. Disoprophylophosphofluoridate (DIPF), one of these agents, reacts with a critical serine residue at the active site on the enzyme to form an inactive diisopropylphosphoryl enzyme :

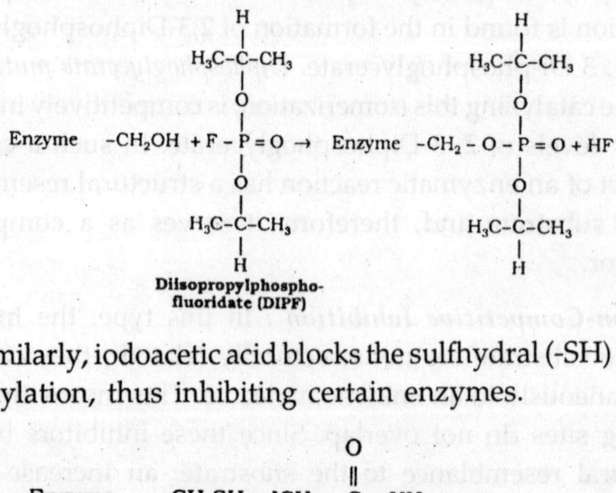

Diisopropylphospho-fluoridate (DIPF)

Similarly, iodoacetic acid blocks the sulfhydral (-SH) groups by alkylation, thus inhibiting certain enzymes.

$$\text{Enzyme} \; -CH_2SH + \underbrace{ICH_2 - \overset{O}{\overset{\|}{C}} - NH_2}_{\textbf{Iodoacetamide}} \longrightarrow$$

$$\text{Enzyme} \; -CH_2 - S - CH_2 - \overset{O}{\overset{\|}{C}} - NH_2 + HI$$

Other examples of irreversible inhibition are the inhibition of many enzymes by heavy metal ions such as Ag^+ Hg^{2+} and Pb^{2+} etc. *Urease* is extremely sensitive to traces of these ions.

Allosteric Enzymes

The kinetic properties of many enzymes cannot be accounted for by the Michaelis-Menten model. An important group consists of the *allosteric enzymes* which usually exhibit sigmoidal rather than hyperbolic plots of the reaction velocity V, versus substrate concentration [S]. They are *oligomers* containing two *(dimer)*, four *[tetramer)*, or more subunits which are able to interact with one another. In allosteric enzymes, one active site in an enzyme molecule can affect another active site in the same enzyme molecule. Due to this interaction across subunits, the binding of the substrate becomes cooperative, which would give a sigmoidal plot of V versus [S].

The sigmoidal shape of the curve results from the fact that the binding of the *first* substrate molecule increases the affinity for binding the *second* substrate molecule, and so forth. Allosteric enzymes are of great regulatory value, since large changes in activity can be obtained by small change in substrate concentration [S]. They are of utmost importance in the regulation of cell metabolism.

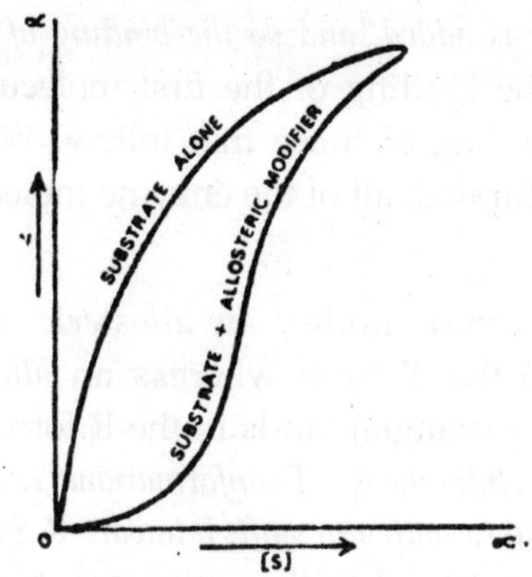

Two models have been postulated to account for some properties of allosteric enzymes. They are (1) the *concerted model* and (2) the *sequential model.*

***The Concerted Model for Allosteric Interactions*:** According to this model proposed in 1965 by Monod, Wyman and Changeux, an allosteric enzyme is made up of two identical subunits, each with one active site. A subunit can exist in either of two conformational states, called R and T. R has a high affinity for the substrate whereas T has a low affinity. Forms R and T are interconvertible. An important supposition of this model is that both subunits must be in the same conformational state, in order that the symmetry of the dimer is conserved. Thus RR and TT are permissible conformations, but RT is not allowed.

In the absence of substrate, most of the enzyme molecules are in the T form. Since the substrate binds preferentially to the R form, the addition of substrate shifts the conformational equilibrium in the direction of the R form when substrate binds to one site, the other site on the same enzyme molecule must also be in the R form, according to the basic concept of this model. It could be said, therefore, that the transition from T to R or vice versa is concerted or arranged. In this way, *the proportion of enzyme molecules in the R form increases progressively as more substrate is added, and so the binding of the substrate is cooperative i.e.,* the binding of the first molecule of substrate enhances the binding of those that follow. When the active sites are fully saturated, all of the enzyme molecules are in the R form.

In the concerted model, an *allosteric inhibitor* binds preferentially to the T form whereas an *allosteric activator* (represented by a triangle) binds to the R form. Therefore, *an allosteric inhibitor shifts the R = T conformational equilibrium toward* T, *whereas an allosteric activator shifts it toward R.* Such modulators or modifiers do not bind to the active site, but to a different site-the allosteric one.

Allosteric interactions between identical *ligands* are homotropic as in the cooperative binding of substrate to the enzyme. Homo-tropic interactions are *necessarily positive* in the concerted model. Interactions between different ligands are referred to as heterotropic. For example, the effect of an activator or inhibitor on the binding of substrate is heterotropic because it involves interactions between different kinds of molecules. Heterotropic effects can be either *positive* or *negative.*

Sequential Model for Allosteric Interaction : Allosteric interactions can also be explained by the sequential model which has been developed by Koshland, Nemethy and Filmer. It is based on three assumptions :

(i) Any one subunit can exist in only two conformational states R and T.

(ii) The binding of substrate to one of the subunits induces a change in its conformation, However, the conformation of the other subunits in this enzyme molecule does not change.

(iii) The conformational change induced by the binding of substrate in one subunit can increase or decrease the substrate binding affinity of the other subunits in the same enzyme molecule.

The sequential model differs from the concerted model in many ways :

(1) An equilibrium between the R and T forms in the absence of substrate is not assumed. On the contrary, the conformational change-over from T to R is induced by the binding of substrate.

(2) The conformational change from T to R in different subunits of an enzyme molecule is sequential, not concerted *Ie.,* arranged or adjusted.

(3) The hybrid form RT is prominent in the sequential model but it does not exist in the concerted model.

(4) The concerted model assumes that symmetry is essential

for the interaction of subunits in oligomeric proteins and, therefore requires that it should be conserved in allosteric interactions.

(5) Homotropic interactions are always positive in the concerted model but can be either positive or negative in the sequential model.

The most studied allosteric enzyme is *aspartate transcarbamylase* (ATCase) which catalyzes the conversion of carbamyl phosphate to carbamyl aspartate, the first of a sequence of eight reactions leading to the synthesis of Cytidine Triphosphate (CTP), which, in turn, is required for the synthesis of the nucleic acids. This is illustrated in the following equations:

$$\text{Carbamyl phosphate} \xrightarrow{\text{At Case}} \text{Carbamyl aspartate} \overset{\text{7 Steps}}{\cdots\cdots\rightarrow} \text{CTP} \cdots\cdots \rightarrow \text{Nucleic acids}$$

When CTP begins to accumulate as a result of a decrease in the rate of nucleic acid synthesis within the cell, it reaches a concentration which makes it an inhibitor of AT Case, thereby inhibiting its own synthesis. This effect is termed negative feed back control.

The enzyme AT Case consists of 12 subunits equally divided among two kinds : six subunits of A, and six of B. Subunits A contain binding sites for the substrate, carbamyl phosphate, but do not bind CTP ; they contain the catalytic sites. Subunits B bind CTP and lack catalytic activity. The binding site for CTP is termed the allosteric site (allo= Other) ; such an enzyme is called an allosteric enzyme, and the inhibition is called allosteric inhibition.

Coenzymes

"Coenzymes generally act as acceptors or donors of a functional group or of atoms that are removed from or contributed to the substrate." Types of reactions that frequently require the participation of coenzymes are oxidoreductions, group transfer, isomerization reactions and reactions resulting in the formation of covalent such as those catalyzed by the enzymes of the digestive tract, are not known to require coenzymes.

The majority of coenzymes are chemical derivatives of nucleotides. In most coenzymes, the nitrogen-base portion of nucleotides is replaced by another chemical unit. This unit is usually a derivative of a B vitamin.

Thus many enzymes concerned with the metabolism of amino acids require enzymes containing vitamin B_6 or *pyridoxine.* The B vitamins *nicotinamide, thiamin, riboflavin, pantothenicacid,* and *lipoicacid* are important constituents of coenzymes for biological redox reactions. Similarly *folic acid* and *cobamide* coenzymes function in one-carbon metabolism.

Classification of Coenzymes Based on Functional Characteristics

(A) Coenzymes for transfer of H

S.No.	*Coenzyme*	*Function*	*Essential nutritional factor of vitamin*
1.	Nicotinamide adenine dinucleotide (NaD^+)	Hydrogen Carrier	Nicotinic acid
2.	Nicotinamide adenine dinucleotide phosphate ($NADP^+$)	Hydrogen Carrier	Nicotinic acid
3.	Flavin mononucleotide (FMN)	Hydrogen Carrier	Riboflavin
4.	Flavin adinine dinucleotide (FAD)	Hydrogen Carrier	Riboflavin
5.	Lipoic acid	Hydrogen Carrier	None
6.	Coenzymes Q (Ubiquinone)— An important component of the ETS in the mitochondria	Hydrogen Carrier	None

In older literature, *nicotinamide adenine dinucleotide (NAD$^+$)* is also called *diphosphopyridine nucleotide (DPN$^+$)* or *coenzyme* I. Similarly *nicotinamide adenine dinucleotide phosphate (NADP$^+$)* is called *triphosphopyridine nucleotide (TPN)* or *coenzyme II.*

Because DPN$^+$ is not a nucleotide of 'diphosphopyridine', because this name does not indicate the presence either of nicotinamide or adenine, and because this nomenclature is not in keeping with that used for many related compounds, an International Commission on Nomenclature in 1961 suggested that these two coenzymes be designated as *nicotinamide adenine dinucleotide (NAD)* and *nicotinamide adenine dinucleotide-phosphate (NADP)*. Their reduced forms in this convention, are denoted as NADH, and NADPH, respectively.

(i) NAD$^+$ consists of 2 nucleotide units : *nicotinamide mononucleotide* (NMN: nicotinamide-ribose-O-P), derived from the dietary supply of nicotinamide; and *adenosine monophosphate* (AMP : adenine-ribose-O-P).

(ii) NADP$^+$ is essentially identical with that of NAD$^+$, except that it possess in addition a phosphate ester group attached to the 2'-hydroxyl group of the ribose portion of the adenesine unit.

(iii) FMN is a metabolically active form of the vitamin riboflavin (B_2) to which in cells, a phosphate group becomes linked.

(iv) FAD comprises two nucleotides : FMN and AMP.

Functions : Vitamin B derived coenzymes as mentioned above are capable of being reversibly oxidised and reduced. They are associated with essentially all of the oxidation and reduction reactions occurring within living cells.

They serve as carriers in many processes in which hydrogen is transferred from one compound to another.

(B) Coenzymes for Group Transfer of Groups other than H.

S.No.	*Coenzyme*	*Function*	*Nutrient factor or Essential Vitamin*
1.	ATP and its relatives	Transphosphorylation	None
2.	Coenzyme A (CoA)	Acetyl of other acyl group transfer ; fatty acid synthesis and oxidation.	Pantothenic acid
3.	Thiamin pyrophosphate (Cocarboxylase)	Oxidative decarboxylation of α -keto acids; active aldehyde carrier.	Thiamin
4.	Pyridoxal phos-phate	Reactions involving amino acids *e.g.*, decarboxylation, transmination.	Pyridoxine
5.	Tetrahydrofolic acid	Reactions involving one carbon compounds.	Folic acid
6.	Biotin	CO_2 transfer.	Biotin
7.	Cobamide coenzymes	Carbon chain isomerizations and certain -CH_3 group transfers.	Cyanacobalamin (B_{12})
8.	Lipoic acid	Oxidative decarboxylation acyl acceptor.	

Coenzymes A : A molecule of this compound consists of three parts :

A phosphate derivative + Pantothenic acid (a B vitamin) + A chain of N, C and S atoms to which H is attached.

CoA serves as a carrier of a molecular group called *acetyl,* a 2-carbon unit of importance in respiration and synthesis. An acetyl group gets attached to the S end of the CoA, and the product *acetyl CoA,* is held together by an - S ~ C bond. Like the O ~ P bond, the - S ~ C bond is also a high energy bond. Thus CoA may be considered to be both an acetyl carrier and an energy carrier.

CoA was discovered by the American Biochemist Dr. Fritz Lipmann for which he got the Nobel Prize in 1955.

Since coenzymes are frequently readily dissociable from the enzyme protein, they may properly be regarded as second substrates or *cosubstrates.* This is so for 2 reasons :

1. The chemical changes in the coenzymes exactly counter balance those taking place in the substrate *e.g.* in transphosphorylation reactions involved in the metabolism of sugars, for every molecule of sugar phosphorylated, one molecule of ATP is dephosphorylated and converted to ADP.

   $$\text{ATP} + \text{Sugar} \longrightarrow \text{Sugar-phosphate} + \text{ADP}$$

   Similarly in oxidoreduction (dehydrogenase) reactions, one molecule of substrate is oxided (dehydrogenated) and one molecule of coenzyme is reduced (hydrogenated).

2. A second reason to give equal importance to the reactions of the coenzyme is that this aspect of the reaction may actually be of greater fundamental physiological significance. For example, without NAD^+ glycolysis cannot continue and anaerobic ATP synthesis ceases.

Isoenzymes

An enzyme which has multiple molecular forms in the same organism catalyzing the same reaction is called an *isoenzyme.* Isoenzymes are physically distinct forms of the same catalytic activity. Thus they catalyze the same chemical reaction. Isoenzymes of a particular enzyme are analogous to 10-paisa coins minted at several different mints *e.g.*, at Calcutta, Poona, Madras etc.

The monetary value (reaction catalyzed $\rightleftharpoons$ biologic value) is identical in each instance, and each coin (isoenzyme) is physically quite similar. But just like "mint marks" on a coin, minute physical, chemical and immunological differences between isoenzymes become apparent on careful examination.

The best studied isoenzyme is *Lactic dehydrogenase* (LDH) which can occur in 5 possible forms in the blood sera and tissues of most vertebrates. Two basically different types of LDH occur :

Heart LDH : It occurs in the heart and consists of 4 identical H subunits, *viz.*, HHHH.

Muscle LDH : It is present in the skeletal muscles and consists of 4 similar M subunits, *viz.*, MMMM.

Only the tetrameric molecule possesses catalytic activity. Synthesis of two subunits H and M have been shown to be controlled by distinct genetic loci. Combinations of H and M subunits will produce three additional types of hybrid enzymes. The possible combinations of the H and M subunits are as follows :

Lactate Dehydrogenase Isoenzyme	***Subunits***
I_1	HHHH
I_2	HHHM
I_3	HHMM
I_4	HMMM
I_5	MMMM

There are more than 100 enzymes which are known to exist as isoenzymes. Isoenzymes of numerous dehydrogenases, and of several oxidases, transaminases, phosphatases, transphosphorylases and proteolytic enzymes have been reported. It is now well established that these isoenzymes are produced by genetic changes that determine differences in the amino acid sequence.

Enzymes and Enzyme Activity : One of the most important functions of proteins in living cells is to act as enzymes. The word "enzyme" was first introduced by *Kuhne* in 1878. It is derived from the original Greek word *enzyme* (Gr. *en* = in + *zyme* = leaven), which means *"in yeast"*. In 1896, *Buchner* succeeded in extracting from the yeast cells' a substance that was as active in fermentation as the original yeast. This substance was later called *zymase* and represents a part of the enzyme system involved in fermentation. Thus, our early knowledge about enzymes is based on yeast cells. In 1926, Professor *J.B.Sumner* of Cornell University isolated from jack beans, by means of acetone, the enzyme *urease* in crystalline form. The isolation of the first enzyme in crystalline form was a key discovery for which Prof. Sumner was awarded the Nobel Prize in 1946. Since then investigators have isolated a large number of enzymes and the study of enzymes *(Enzymology)* has its own place in modern Biology, Biochemistry and Physiology.

Definition : *An enzyme may be defined as a complex biological catalyst that is produced by a living organism in its cells to regulate the various physiological processes of the body.*

The substance on which an enzyme acts is called the "substrate". A catalyst is any organic or inorganic substance that accelerates a chemical reaction without affecting the end products of the reaction and without being destroyed in the course of the reaction. All chemical reactions occurring in living cells, and therefore all metabolic processes are mediated by the highly specific biological catalysts, called enzymes. Thus, it can be safely assumed that there must be thousands of enzymes in the animal body, for practically all physiological processes are mainly enzymatic.

Enzymes are involved in such biological processes as digestion, respiration, the stepwise breaking down, synthesis, and inter-conversion of carbohydrates, fats, proteins and nucleic acids, and the release and utilization of energy by the living cells. However, a few protoplasmic activities such as the secretion of milk by mammary glands may involve no enzymes.

Enzymes as Biological Catalysts : Enzymes act as catalysts and are very effective in small amounts. For instance, a single molecule of *catalase*, the enzyme that splits hydrogen peroxide (H_2O_2) into oxygen and water, can effectively transform more than 5 million hydrogen peroxide molecules a minute at certain temperatures. This reaction is shown below :

$$2H_2O_2 \xrightarrow{Catalase} 2H_2O + O_2$$

However, other enzymes are not as effective , but many of them can split up to 500,000 molecules of the substrate per minute.

In the case of *urease,* the enzyme that catalyses the reaction of urea with water, the rate of enzymatic reaction can be speeded up by a factor of 10^{14} over the uncatalyzed reaction. We call the absolute rate in optimum conditions as the ***turnover number*** of the enzyme, the number of reactions catalyzed by the enzyme per second. Urease has a turnover number of 10^4/sec. *i.e.,* one enzyme molecule will catalyze the hydrolysis of 10,000 urea molecules per second. Biological catalysis by enzymes obeys the same general rules observed for non-enzymatic catalysis. That is, enzymes:

1. are effective in very small concentrations.
2. are unchanged by the reaction.
3. exert their physiological effects by changing the rate at which equilibrium is reached, not by changing the equilibrium of the reaction.

Enzymes as biological catalysts differ from other forms of catalysts in the following respects:

(i) Enzymes are highly specific because each enzyme usually catalyzes one particular kind of reaction, whereas a non-biological catalyst (organic or inorganic), such as finely divided platinum, catalyzes a wide variety of reactions.

(ii) All enzymes, consist entirely or in part, of specific proteins which account for their extraordinary degree of specificty that they exhibit.

(iii) Enzymes have greater effectiveness in lowering the activation energy barrier, *i.e.,* lowering the activation energy requirement speeds up the rate dramatically during enzyme catalysis, because a greater fraction of the substrate molecules has sufficient energy to form the activated complex and can, therefore, react.

Chemical Nature of Enzymes : All enzymes are proteins with large molecular weights. Many of them, such as pepsin (a digestive enzyme), are pure proteins made up of chains of amino acids. Others, such as certain vitamins, consist of protein plus some other type of non-protein organic compound. On the basis of differences in chemical nature, the enzymes may be described as follows :

(1) *Apoenzymes and Coenzymes* : Digestive enzymes, such as pepsin and trypsin, are made up entirely of protein, but many others have two parts : a protein part called the *apoenzyme* (Greek *apo*, away from) and a non-protein part, called the *co-factor*. The combination of the two can be referred to as the *enzyme system*. There can be an enzymatic activity only when both components (apoenzyme and co-factor) are present together.

Neither of the two can produce catalytic action by itself. This relation may be shown as :

apoenzyme + cofactor $\longrightarrow$ holoenzyme (or active enzyme)

The cofactor is sometimes a simple divalent metallic ion (*e.g.*, Ca, Mg, Zn, Co, etc.), and sometimes a non-protein organic compound. However, some enzymes require both kinds of cofactors. If the cofactor is firmly bound to the apoenzyme, it is called *prosthetic group* (Gr. *prosthesis,* in addition). For example, cytochromes are the enzymes that possess *porphyrins* as their prosthetic groups. If, instead of being more or less permanently bound to the apoenzyme, the cofactor attaches itself to the apoenzyme only at the time of reaction, it is called a *coenzyme.*

(ii) *Metalloenzymes* : Numerous enzymes contain small quantities of a particular metallic ion in their make-up and are accordingly called *metalloenzymes.* For example, the ions of magnesium, calcium, phosphate, copper, zinc or iron, etc., may be the specific metal components of particular enzymes. The presence of the metal is usually necessary for enzymatic activity, and its removal causes a loss in the catalytic action of the enzyme. In modern enzymology, these simple substances (metallic ions), closely associated with the protein of the enzyme of which they are also a part, are called by *Bersin* as *compliments.* However, some enzymes are composed not only of a specific protein but of a coenzyme and a metallic component or activator as well.

(iii) *Isozymes* : An enzyme which has multiple molecular forms in the same organism is known as an *isozyme.* The most thoroughly studied isozyme is *lactic dehydrogenase* (LDH) which can occur in five possible forms in organs of most vertebrates as observed by careful starch gel electrophoretic separation. Two basically different types of LDH occur. One type, which is inhibited strongly by relatively low concentrations of pyruvate, predominates in the heart and is called the *heart LDH.* The other type, less easily inhibited by pyruvate, occurs in many skeletal muscles and is thus called the *muscle LDH.* The heart enzyme consists of 4 identical sub-units, which are called H sub-units. The muscle enzyme consists of 4 identical M sub-units. The two types of sub-units, H and M, have different amino acid compositions and have different immunological properties. There is genetic evidence that two sub-units are produced by two separate genes.

Source and Site of Action of Enzymes : All enzymes are formed inside the living cell. On the basis of the site of their action, they may be called as follows :

(i) *Endoenzymes* : Enzymes which normally act only within the cells (intracellular) are called *endoenzymes* and are represented by such an enzyme as *cytochrome oxidase.* This respiratory enzyme was discovered by *Warburg* in 1926. It catalyses the oxidation of cytochromes by oxygen for, in the presence of free oxygen and cytochrome oxidase, cytochrome gives up its hydrogen to the oxygen with the formation of water.

(ii) *Exoenzymes* : Enzymes which normally work after they have been secreted by the cells are called extracellular or *exoenzymes.* They perform their work in secretions such as the digestive enzymes.

Physical Properties of Enzymes : Most of the enzymes are colourless, but some are brown, red or green, etc. Most of them are generally soluble in water, but those with lipoprotein are insoluble in water. All are insoluble in absolute alcohol and most of them are destroyed or made inactive by temperatures over 65°C. Enzymes are colloidal in nature and behave like colloids with a precipitation agent.

Functional Properties of Enzymes : The main functional properties of the enzymes are as follows :

1. An enzyme is a protein molecule with one or more active sites and it catalyzes or speeds up a reaction.
2. The enzyme works at extremely small concentrations. Because enzyme appears unchanged at the end of the reaction, very small amount of the enzyme used over and over again can catalyse very large quantities of substrates.

3. From thermodynamic point of view an enzyme is a catalytic agent which speeds up a reaction by *lowering the activation energy*. It does so by increasing the number of molecules that are activated and therefore reactive.
4. Being a protein, an enzyme loses its catalytic properties if subjected to agents like heat, strong acids or bases, organic solvents, or other materials, which denature the protein.
5. The enzyme activity is influenced by temperature, pH, concentration of enzyme, and substrate concentration.
6. Each enzyme usually acts on a single substrate. This is known as specificity of enzyme action.
7. Some enzymes exist as *proenzymes*, which are inactive and their activation is necessary to catalyse a reaction.
8. The rate of an enzyme catalyzed reaction may be decreased by a substance, which is known as inhibitor, and the phenomenon is described as enzyme inhibition.
9. A particular enzyme is effective in accelerating a reaction in either direction, for it does not determine the direction of a reaction.

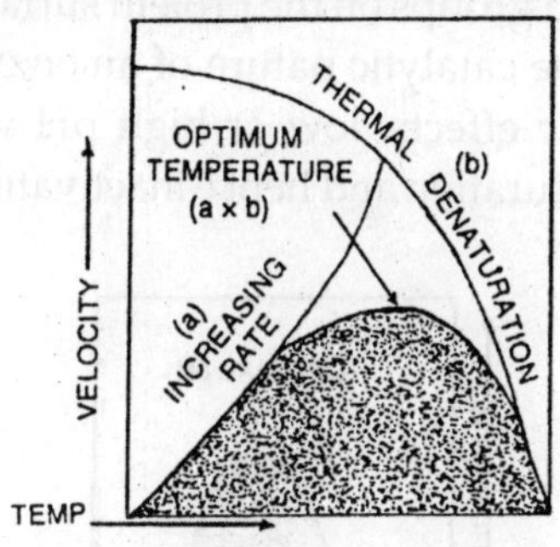

Effect of temperature on reaction rate of an enzyme catalysed reaction. (a) represents the increasing rate of a reaction as a function of temp, (b) represents the decreasing rate as a function of thermal denaturation of the enzyme protein. The shaded area represents the combination of a×b.

Effect of Temperature on Enzyme Action : As temperature rises, the effectiveness of an enzyme increases up to a certain *optimum* level but decreases thereafter. The temperature at which an enzyme works its best is known as the *temperature optimum* (Fig.). Though each particular type of enzyme has its own specific temperature optimum, most enzymes operate optimally in a temperature range of about 25 to 40°C. At lower than optimal temperatures enzymes are less effective, primarily, because reactions of all kinds decrease in rate in a colder environment, and at higher than optimal temperatures the physical structure of the enzyme proteins begins to be destroyed. The *thermal denaturation* of the enzyme protein, thus, decreases the effective concentration of an enzyme, and consequently decreases the reaction rate.

Effect of pH on Enzyme Action

The pH at which maximum enzyme activity occurs varies considerably from one enzyme to another. This is known as the *pH optimum* (Fig.). For example, digestive enzyme *pepsin* has an optimum activity at pH_2. But many other enzymes work in a pH range of 6 to 7.5 or more. Since enzymes are proteins, pH-changes normally affect the ionic character of the amino and carboxylic acid groups on the protein surface and therefore, markedly affect the catalytic nature of an enzyme. In addition to the purely ionic effects, low or high pH values can cause considerable denaturation and hence inactivation of the enzyme protein.

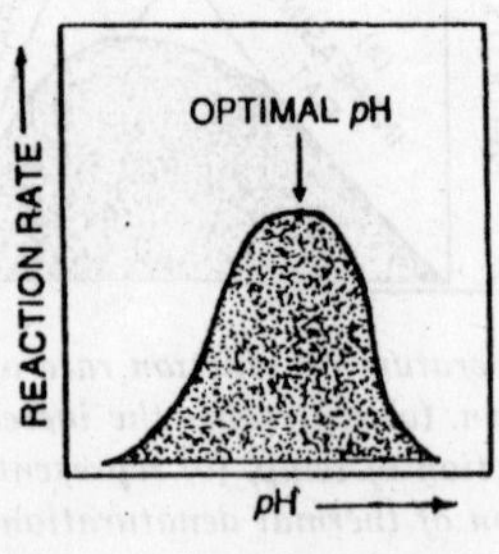

Effect of pH on an enzyme-catalyzed reaction.

Effect of Enzyme Concentration on Enzyme Action : The rate of an enzyme-catalysed reaction depends directly on the *concentration of the enzyme,* assuming that substrate concentration is in saturating amounts. The effect of enzyme on reaction rate can be appreciated by considering the *turnover number* of an enzyme. It is the number of moles of substrate converted to product per minute per mole of enzyme (when the enzyme is fully saturated with substrate). For example, *amylase,* an enzyme involved in the breakdown of starch and other polysaccharides, has a turnover number of 10×10^5, *i.e.,* it can hydrolyse about 10^5 glycosidic bonds per minute and no detectable hydrolysis occurs in the absence of amylase. Urease has a turnover number of 10^4/sec, *i.e.,* one enzyme molecule will catalyze the hydrolysis of 10,000 urea molecules per second. The turnover numbers of most enzymes fall between 10^2 and 10^6.

Effect of Substrate Concentration on Enzyme Action : The effect of substrate concentration on enzyme action was first studied independently by *Henri* and *Brown* (1902) showing the action of invertase on sucrose :

$$\text{Sucrose} + \text{invertase} \rightarrow \text{Sucrose-invertase} \rightarrow \text{glucose} + \text{fructose} + \text{invertase}$$

Thus, *V. Henri* (1902) was the first to suggest that the enzyme and substrate combine with each other. Therefore, at high substrate concentrations, the rate of enzyme-catalyzed reaction becomes limited by the enzyme concentration, which is held constant in various reactions.

The first satisfactory mathematical analysis of the effect of substrate concentration on the reaction velocity of enzyme-catalysed reaction was made by *Michaelis* and *Menten* (1913). With fixed enzyme concentration, an increase of substrate will result at first in a very rapid rise in the velocity or reaction rate. As the substrate concentration continues to increase, however, the increase in the rate of reaction begins to slow down until, with a large substrate concentration, no further change in the velocity is observed. The velocity of the reaction obtained at this high substrate concentration is defined as the *maximum velocity* (Vm) of the enzyme-catalyzed reaction under the specified conditions (Fig.) and the initial reaction velocity obtained with substrate concentrations below the saturation level is called *v.*

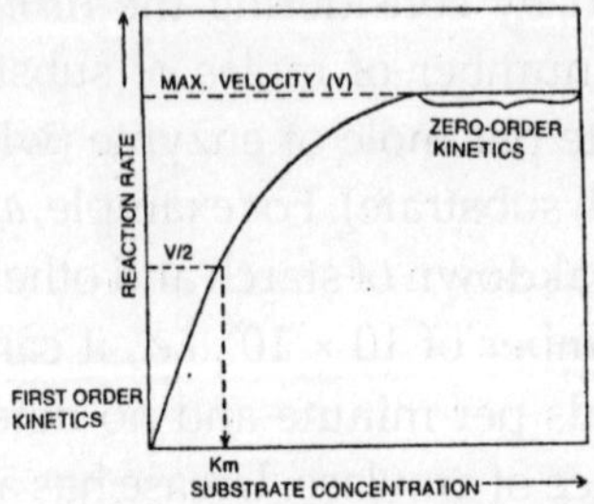

The effect of substrate concentration on reaction rate, assuming that the enzyme concentration is constant.

The substrate concentration required to yield half the maximum velocity (Vm/2) can be readily determined from Fig., and is an important constant in the enzyme chemistry. It defines the *Michaelis constant* or Km. In other words, Km is defined as the substrate concentration when v= 1/2 Vm. Under carefully defined conditions of temperature, pH, and ionic strength of the buffer, this constant Km approximates the dissociation constant of an enzyme-substrate complex. The reciprocal of Km or 1/Km, approximates the affinity of an enzyme for its substrate. Thus, a Km of 0.1 mole/1 of substrate would indicate that the active site of an enzyme is half saturated, when its substrate is present at that concentration. The enzyme, therefore, has a low affinity for its substrate. On the other hand, a Km of 0.0001 mole/1 indicates that the enzyme has a high affinity, since it is half saturated at this low substrate concentration.

Kinetics of Enzyme Action

The Michaelis constant (Km) is of considerable importance since it provides a valuable clue to the mode of action of an enzyme catalyzing a reaction. It should be noted that at low substrate concentration the relation of velocity to substrate is almost linear and obeys the *first-order kinetics, i.e.,* the rate of the reaction $A \rightarrow B$ is directly proportional to the substrate concentration [A]:

$$v = k' [A] \text{ low [substrate]}$$

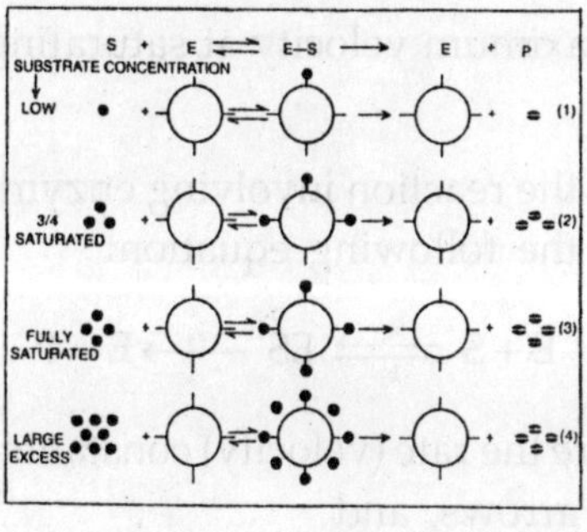

Diagrammatic demonstration of the effect of substrate concentration on saturation of active sites on enzyme surface. Note that for a unit time interval cases 3 and 4 give the same amount of P (product) despite a large excess of substrate in case 4.

where v is the observed velocity of the reaction at concentration [A] and k' is the specific rate constant. At high substrate concentration, however, the velocity of the reaction is maximum and is independent of the substrate [A]; hence it obeys the zero-order kinetics (Fig.).

$$Vm = k' \text{ saturating [substrate]}$$

According to *Michaelis* and others, an enzyme-catalyzed reaction at varying substrate concentrations is *diphasic i.e.,* at low substrate concentrations the active sites on the enzyme are not saturated by the substrate and thus the enzyme is not working at full capacity. As the number of substrate molecules increases, the sites are covered to a great degree till at saturation no more sites are available and the enzyme is working at full capacity. This relationship is shown in Fig., and its mathematical expression *(Michaelis-Menten equation)* is as follows :

$$v = \frac{Vm\,[S]}{Km + [S]} \quad \text{or} \quad Km = [S]\,\frac{Vm - v}{v}$$

where v = initial reaction velocity at given substrate concentration [S],

Km = Michaelis constant, moles /litre

Vm = maximum velocity at saturating concentrations of substrate.

Considering the reaction involving enzyme, substrate, and product we get the following equation:

$$E + S \underset{k_2}{\overset{k_1}{\rightleftharpoons}} ES \xrightarrow{k_3} E + P$$

where k_1, k_2, k_3 are the rate (velocity) constants for the reactions as indicated by arrows, and

$$K_m = (k_2 + k_3)/k_1$$

The Michaelis-Menten equation is useful for the following purposes :

1. It allows us to calculate the degree of saturation of an enzyme at a given substrate concentration. At the concentration of substrate equal to Km, the enzyme is half-saturated.
2. We can determine Km and Vm for an impure enzyme preparation in which the concentration or even the amount of enzyme is not known. Typically, the Km will be the same as for the pure enzyme but Vm can be expressed only in specific enzyme units—the number of micromoles of product formed per minute per milligram of the enzyme protein.
3. If the molar concentration of catalytic sites is known, then we can calculate the *turnover number* (the number of substrate molecules changed into product per enzyme molecule per second) when the enzyme is fully saturated.

4. It permits to compare the kinetics of a given enzyme with respect to a variety of substrates.

5. It helps identify regulatory enzymes which do not strictly obey classical Michaelis-Menten kinetics.

6. Km and Vm are also important from the point of view of cell metabolism. An enzyme cannot catalyze a reaction that uses a substrate whose concentration is very much lower than the value of Km. Cellular metabolism has presumably evolved to keep Km in proper relation to substrates. Similarly, an enzyme cannot catalyze a reaction faster than Vm. When the reaction product is needed at a faster rate, more enzymes must be synthesized (Loewy *et al*, 1991).

Specificity of Enzyme Action

The protein nature of the enzyme confers on the enzyme the property of *specificity i.e.,* each enzyme usually acts on a single substrate or a group of closely related substrates. However, the degree of specificity of enzymes is variable. In some cases it is *absolute,* and in others, it is *relative.* The various kinds of specificity exhibited by enzymes are as follows :

Absolute Reaction Specificity : In this case only one type of reaction is catalyzed. For example, hydrolysis of fumaric acid into L-malic acid by *fumarase;* hydration of CO_2 to carbonic acid by *carbonic anhydrase,* etc.

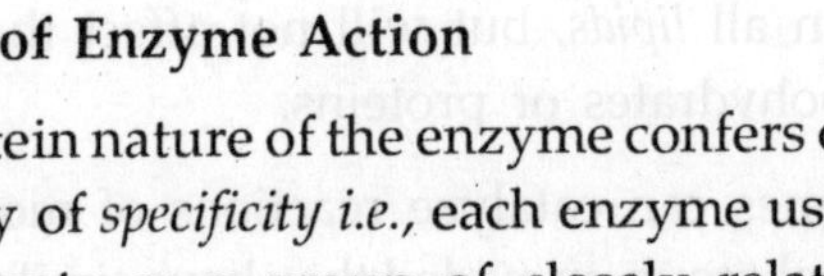

Absolute Substrate Specificity : In this case the enzyme acts on only one substrate. For example, *urease* can utilize only *urea* as a substrate and will fail to act an even the slightest chemical modification of urea.

$$\underset{\text{Urea}}{NH_2{-}\overset{O}{\overset{\|}{C}}{-}NH_2} + H_2O \xrightarrow{urease} 2NH_3 + CO_2$$

$$\underset{\text{Biuret}}{NH_2{-}\overset{O}{\overset{\|}{C}}{-}NH{-}\overset{O}{\overset{\|}{C}}{-}NH_2} + H_2O \xrightarrow{urease} \text{no reaction}$$

Group Specificity **:** In this case enzymes act on compounds possessing a particular chemical group. The enzyme *alcohol dehydrogenase* exhibits such group specificity. There is a strong requirement for the (OH) group, which is oxidised to an aldehyde

$$CH_3CH_2OH + \underset{\text{co-enzyme}}{\text{Oxidized}} \xrightleftharpoons{\text{alcohol dehydrogenase}} \underset{+\ \text{reduced co-enzyme}}{CH_3CHO}$$

Although ethanol is probably the natural substrate, alcohol dehydrogenase can also act on straight chain alcohols of similar lenghts. Similarly, *lipase* will catalyse the rupture of a specific chemical link in all *lipids,* but will not affect that linkage if present in carbohydrates or proteins.

Some enzymes can catalyze reactions of more than one kind of functional group, provided they have similar structures. Such *relative group specificity* is found in the enzyme *trypsin,* which can hydrolyse an *ester* bond as well as a *peptide* bond, but requires a positively charged functional group (side chain of lysine or arginine on the carbonyl (C=O) side of the ester or peptide bond).

Stereo-chemical Specificity **:** In this case the enzymes act on only one optical isomer of a compound. For example, the enzyme *L-amino acid oxidase* will not act on D-amino acids.

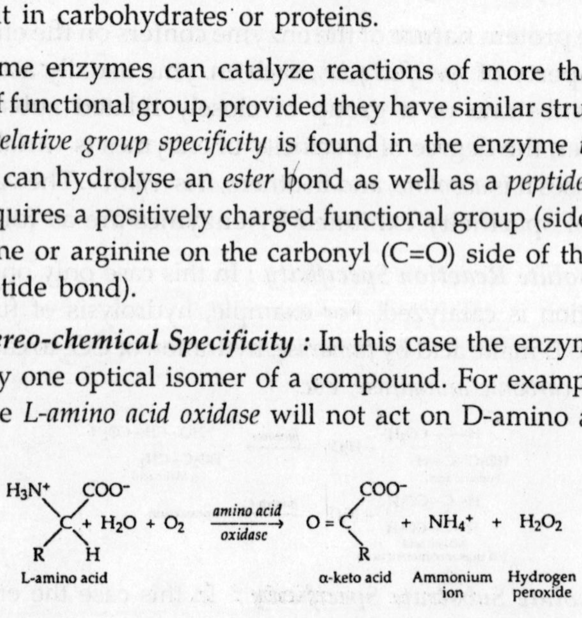

Similarly, D-amino acid oxidase will oxidise D-amino acids only. Stereospecificity can only be explained that there is at least a *three-point contact* between the enzyme active site and the four substituents of the asymmetric carbon atom.

Theories of Enzyme Specificity

Probing enzyme specificity with various chemical compounds thus gives clues about the structure of the *active site,* a special location on the enzyme. It is in binding substrate to the active site that selectivity is exerted. The following theories explain the enzyme-substrate interaction and enzyme specificity.

The lock-and-key Theory : *Emil Fischer* (1894) postulated that an enzyme allows only one or a few compounds to fit onto its surface. This is the lock-and-key hypothesis according to which the enzyme and its substrate have a complementary shape. In other words, the theory proclaims that there is complementary structural relationship of enzyme and substrate. This theory is based on the concept that each enzyme molecule has definite surface configurations into which the substrate fits quite easily just like a key fits into its lock.

The specific substrate molecules are bound to a specific region of the enzyme molecule called its *active site.* The active site of an enzyme is formed by a number of amino acid residues whose side chains have two principal roles : *(a)* they serve to *attract* and *orient* the substrate in a specific manner within the site (such amino acids are called *contact residues* and contribute in large degree to substrate specificity), and *(b)* they participate in the formation of temporary bonds with the substrate molecule, bonds that polarize the substrate, introduce strain into certain of its bonds and trigger the catalytic change (such amino acids are termed *catalytic residues).*

The contact and catalytic residues that make up the active site may be located in widely separated regions of the enzyme's primary structure, but as a result of stabilized polypeptide chain folding, they are brought into the appropriate juxtaposition. This is exemplified by the enzyme *lysozyme* in which the amino acids that form the active site in the folded structure are widely separated in the primary structure. The bonds formed between a substrate and the amino acid side chains forming the active site may be either covalent or non-covalent. The lock-and-key model of enzyme catalysis accounts for enzyme specificity, since compounds that lack the appropriate shape (or are too large or too small) cannot be bound to the active site.

Induced-fit Theory : According to this theory, proposed by *Daniel Koshland* (1963), the active site of the enzyme does not initially exist in a shape that is complementary to the substrate, but is induced to assume the complementary shape as the substrate becomes bound. As *Koshland* put it, the active site is induced to assume complementary shape *"in much the same way as a hand induces a change in the shape of a glove"*. Thus, according to the induced-fit model, the enzyme (or its active site) is *flexible.*

The induced-fit theory is more attractive because the protein molecule is flexible enough to allow conformational changes, and because it allows some explanation for the influence of hormones on enzymatic activity. The induced-fit model explains the effects of certain competitive and non-competitive inhibitors of enzyme action.

Enzyme Activation

Many enzymes are simple proteins and need no additional factor to work at full capacity . However, some of these proteins exist as *proenzymes* or *zymogens,* which are inactive. For example, *trypsinogen, pepsinogen* and *cryptotrypsinogen* are zymogens that have been isolated and carefully studied. To transform the zymogen to an active enzyme an inhibitory or a blocking peptide must be removed. When trypsinogen is converted to trypsin by enterokinase or trypsin, for example, there is a loss of a hexapeptide consisting of valine, aspartic acid, and lysine from the amino terminal end resulting in a change in the conformation of the protein.

$$\text{trypsinogen} \xrightarrow{trypsin} \text{trypsin} + \text{Val (asp)}_4 \text{ lysine}$$

Another type of activation depends on maintaining the integrity of *Sulfhydryl* (—SH) groups in the enzyme protein. These groups may maintain or perhaps constitute part of the active centre of the enzyme. If they are oxidised to disulphide form (—S—S—), the enzyme becomes inactive. For example, proteolytic enzyme *papain* is inert after exposure to O_2. When a suitable reductant is added to convert —S—S— to —SH, papain becomes fully activated (provided the enzyme is protected from O_2). Similar observations have been made with a large number of enzymes including *pyruvic carboxylase* and *triosephosphate dehydrogenase.*

A third type of activation requires the participation of still another factor in addition to the protein molecule. The general term *cofactor* encompasses this activation. Cofactors, however, may be divided into three groups : *(a)* prosthetic groups, *(b)* coenzymes and (c) metal activators.

(a) *Prosthetic group* is usually considered to be a cofactor *firmly bound* to the enzyme protein. Thus, for example, porphyrin moiety of the *haemoprotein peroxidase* and the firmly associated flavin adenine dinucleotide (FAD) in *succinic dehydrogenase* are prosthetic groups.

(b) *A coenzyme* is a particular kind of cofactor, a non-protein organic compound, that attaches itself to the enzyme protein only at the time of reaction. Thus, NAD, NADP, tetrahydrofolic acid and thiamin pyrophosphate are examples of coenzymes.

(c) The *metal activator* group is represented by the requirement of a large number of enzymes for metallic mono or divalent cations, such as K^+, Mn^{2+}, Mg^{2+} Ca^{2+}

or Zn^{2+}. These may be either loosely or firmly bound to an enzyme protein, presumably by chelation with phenolic, amino, phosphoryl, or carboxyl groups.

A fourth type of activation has recently been correlated with a rather large number of enzymes called *regulatory enzymes,* since their activities are altered by rather subtle factors. In general, these enzymes are made up of several sub-units with at least two stereospecifically different non-overlapping receptor sites. One site, the *active site,* binds the substrate and makes possible the catalytic activity of the protein.

The other site binds another compound at its so-called *regulatory* or *allosteric site,* the compound which is bound, is called an *allosteric effector*. In other words, molecules that do not resemble the substrate but bind to the enzyme and exert an effect are called *allosteric* (allo-steric = other shape). Some workers have also used the term *positive effectors* for compounds that increase the rate of the enzymatically catalyzed reaction and *negative effectors* that have the opposite effect. There is good evidence that there is either a change in the quaternary structure of the enzyme protein or a conformational change such as a folding of the protein from an extended into a more globular form.

The active site is accordingly modified and, therefore, the enzyme activity is altered. The allosteric effector does not undergo any chemical change. This type of enzyme inhibition is called *Allosteric enzyme inhibition* or *Allosterism.*

A regulatory enzyme that has been intensively studied is *aspartate transcarbamylase* and its allosteric effector is *cytidylic acid*. Other regulatory enzymes include *phosphofructokinase* which is greatly activated by ADP, muscle *phosphorylase b* activated by 5'-AMP, and *acetyl CoA carboxylase* of mammalian tissues, markedly stimulated by citrate.

Enzyme Inhibition

Substances or compounds that decrease the rate of an enzyme-catalyzed reaction are known as *inhibitors,* and the phenomenon is described as *enzyme inhibition* (Fig.). Inhibitors generally act by combining either with the substrates of the given reaction, making such substrates less reactive at that temperature, or with the enzymes normally required by the given substrates, making such enzymes ineffective. In either case an inhibitor blocks a particular reaction pathway.

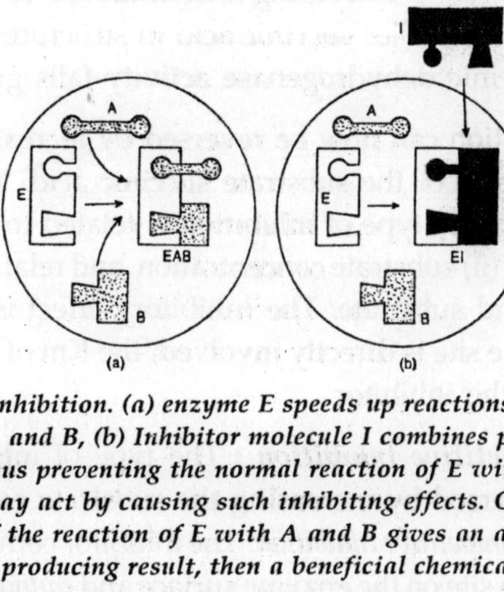

Enzyme Inhibition. (a) enzyme E speeds up reactions involving reactants A and B, (b) Inhibitor molecule I combines preferentially with E, thus preventing the normal reaction of E with A and B. Poisons may act by causing such inhibiting effects. On the other hand, if the reaction of E with A and B gives an abnormal, disease producing result, then a beneficial chemical may be introduced which acts like I and so prevents the disease.

Enzyme inhibition can occur in a variety of ways, and its study can reveal a great deal about the nature of the enzyme and the catalyzed reaction. The following types of enzyme inhibition are known:

Competitive Inhibition **:** When a compound competes with a substrate for the active site on the enzyme protein and thereby reduces the catalytic activity of that enzyme, the compound is considered to be a *competitive inhibitor.* Inhibition by such structural analogues (called *antimeta-*

bolites), which is reversed by simply adding more substrate to the reaction mixture, is known as *competitive inhibition.*

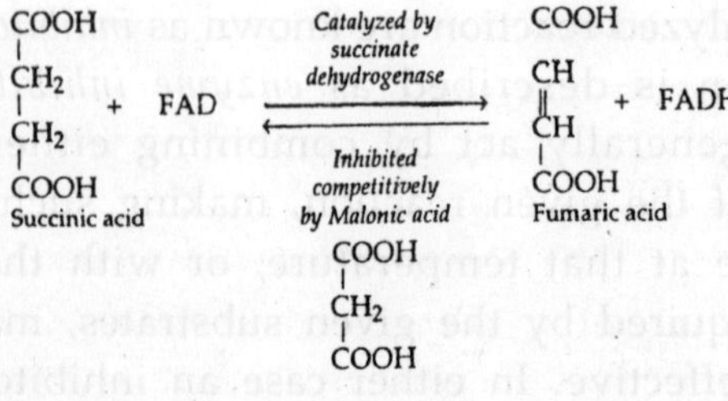

For example, *succinate dehydrogenase* readily oxidises *succinic acid* to *fumaric acid.* If increasing concentrations of *malonic acid,* which closely resembles succinic acid in structure, are added, however, succinic dehydrogenase activity falls greatly.

The inhibition can now be reversed by increasing in turn the concentration of the substrate succinic acid. The amount of inhibition in this type of inhibition is related to (i) inhibitor concentration, (ii) substrate concentration, and relative affinities of inhibitor and substrate. The inhibitory effect is reversible. Since the active site is directly involved, the Km of the enzyme is altered by the inhibitor.

Non-competitive Inhibition : The type of inhibition that cannot be reversed by increasing the substrate concentration is called *non-competitive inhibition.* The inhibitor combines rather strongly with a site on the enzyme surface and *cannot be displaced* by increasing substrate concentration. The amount of inhibition in this type of inhibition is related to (i) inhibitor concentration, and (ii) inhibitor's affinity for the enzyme. The substrate concentration has no effect on this system and the Km is not altered by the inhibitor.

A good example of noncompetitive inhibition is the reaction of iodoacetamide on triose phosphate dehydrogenase, a sulfhydryl enzyme:

$$\text{enzyme - SH} + ICH_2\,CONH_2 \rightarrow \text{enzyme - S - } CH_2\,CONH_2 + HI$$

Feedback (end-product) Inhibition : When end-product of a reaction serves to prevent the formation of one of its own precursors by inhibiting the action of the enzyme catalyzing the very reaction, the inhibition is called *feedback inhibition* .

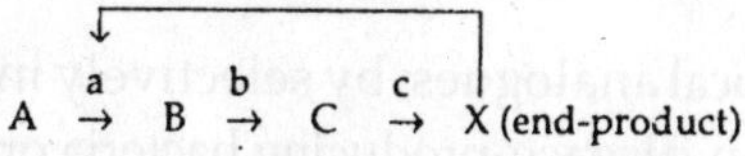

The inhibition of conversion of A to B by X would be such an inhibition. Here X, the ultimate product of the reaction, serves to prevent the formation of one of its own precursors (B) by inhibiting the action of enzyme *a,* which catalyzes the change from A to B . In this instance , enzyme *a* can be called the pacemaker since the entire sequence is effectively regulated by it.

An actual example is the formation of cytidine triphosphate (CTP) from aspartic acid and carbamyl phosphate in *E. coli.* As a critical concentration of CTP is built up, the triphosphate slows down its own formation by inhibiting the enzyme, *aspartate transcarbamylase* (ATC ase), which catalyzes the pacemaker step of its own synthesis. When the concentration of triphosphate is sufficiently lowered by metabolic utilization, inhibition is released, and its synthesis is renewed.

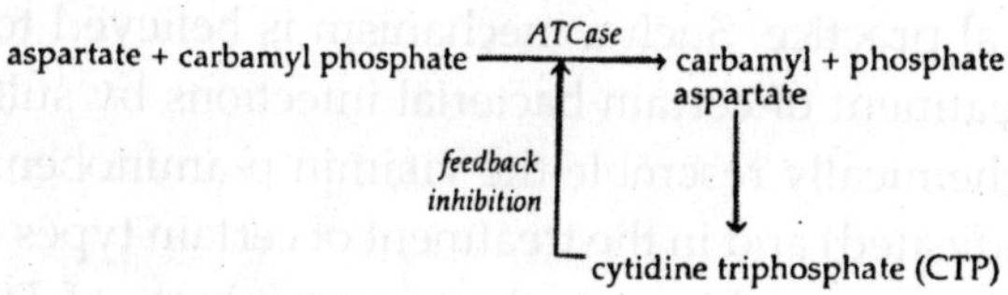

Significance of Inhibition

In living materials inhibitors are of importance in two ways : *An inhibitor blocking a normal reaction represents a disease producing poison, and an inhibitor blocking a disease producing reaction represents a medicinal drug* (Fig.).

The concept of competitive inhibition of enzymes explains

the widely observed competitive effects of various substances, which are structurally related to biologically active compounds. Often minor alterations in the chemical structure of a normal compound may result in a so-called *analogue* that competes with the biologically active material itself.

Some chemical analogues, by selectively inhibiting certain key-enzymes in disease-producing bacteria or cancer cells, can seriously disturb their metabolism, thereby, inhibiting their growth and function without seriously affecting the normal host cells. A well known example of competitive inhibition is the effect of *sulfanilamide* (a sulfa drug), which "fools" the enzyme normally acting on p-aminobenzoic acid, an important growth factor in many bacteria.

The similarity in structure of sulfanilamide and p-aminobenzoic acid is quite apparent.

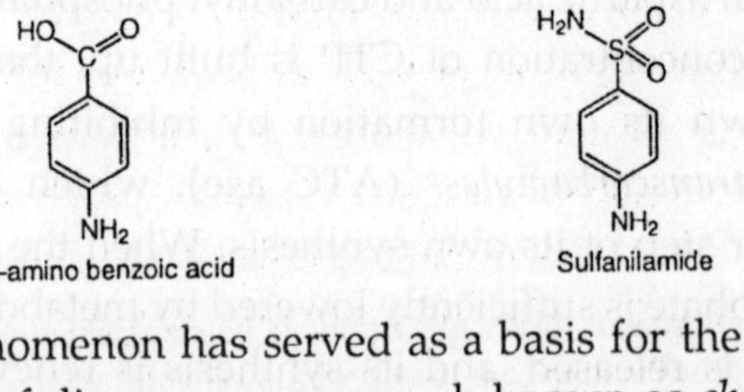

p–amino benzoic acid   Sulfanilamide

This phenomenon has served as a basis for the treatment of a number of diseases, an approach known as *chemotherapy* in medical practice. Such a mechanism is believed to operate in the treatment of certain bacterial infections by sulfa drugs, (which chemically resemble the vitamin p-aminobenzoic acid as just indicated) and in the treatment of certain types of cancer by chemicals resembling the base components of DNA.

The feedback inhibition is responsible for continually adjusting the rate of synthesis of metabolic intermediates according to the demands of synthesis. Usually, an end-product inhibits an early reaction in its synthesis, thereby avoiding the formation of several intermediates, which would be wasteful to the cell.

Reversibility of the Enzyme Action

A particular enzyme is effective in accelerating a reaction in either direction, for it does not determine the direction of a reaction. Thus, most enzymatic reactions are reversible. However, some reversible reactions are of great help in metabolism. For example, in the liver, glucose is converted into glycogen by an enzyme *glycogenase,* and stored up in this form. This happens when there is an excess of glucose in the bloodstream. But when there is a deficiency of glucose in the blood, the same enzyme is capable of reconverting the insoluble glycogen into soluble glucose which then goes to the general bloodstream.

$$\text{Glucose} \xrightleftharpoons{\textit{glycogenase}} \text{Glycogen}$$

Nomenclature and Classification of Enzymes : The most common method of naming enzymes is to add the suffix "ase" to the root word of the substrate on which the enzyme works. Thus, the names of most enzymes end in "ase". For example, *Sucrase* acts upon sucrose, *lipase* upon lipids, *protease* upon proteins, and so on. Some enzymes have special names, such as *pepsin, ptyalin,* and *trypsin,* etc. Sometimes the suffix "lytic" is used in naming enzymes. *Proteolytic* (protein splitting) is a general term for any enzyme that digests protein. The term *amylolytic* (starch splitting), *lipolytic* (fat splitting) and *sucrolytic* (carbohydrate splitting) are used for enzymes that digest starch, fat and carbohydrate respectively.

Enzymes may be conveniently classified into several major groups according to the chemical reactions which they catalyze. Since a chemical reaction catalyzed by an enzyme is the specific property that distinguishes one enzyme from another, six main divisions are employed in the classification of enzymes (as suggested in 1961 in the report of the Commission of Enzymes of the International Union of Biochemistry, I.U.B.)

***Oxidoreductases* :** These are the enzymes which catalyze biological oxidations and reductions—the removal or addition of hydrogen atoms. *Dehydrogenases, Oxidases* (where O_2 acts as acceptor) and *Oxygenases* (where O_2 is partly incorporated into the molecule), and *peroxidases* (where H_2O_2 serves as an acceptor) are the trivial names of the many enzymes found in this class of enzymes. *Malic dehydrogenase* would be given the systematic name of malate-(TPN$^+$) — oxidoreductase.

A dehydrogenase or *reductase* is an enzyme that catalyzes the dehydrogenation or removal of hydrogen atoms (or electrons) from one substrate A, transferring them to another substrate B (other than to molecular O_2).

$$AH_2 + B \xrightarrow{\textit{dehydrogenase}} A + BH_2$$

An *Oxidase* is an enzyme that catalyzes the transfer of hydrogen atoms (or electrons) from a substrate to the molecular O_2 specifically. The O_2 is usually reduced to form water.

$$AH_2 + 1/2\ O_2 \xrightarrow{\textit{Oxidase}} A + H_2O$$

An important oxidoreductase is *lactic acid dehydrogenase,* which catalyzes the following reaction.

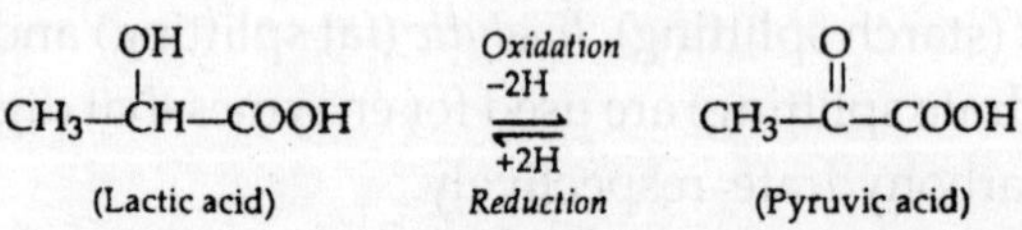

However, in order to perform a catalytic reaction dehydrogenases require specific coenzymes and, in fact, it is the coenzyme that accepts or donates the hydrogen atoms. Nicotinamide adenine dinucleotide (NAD) and NAD phosphate (NADP) are examples of these coenzymes.

***Transferases* :** These are the enzymes that catalyze the transfer of a chemical group from one molecule to another , *e.g., transaminases, transphosphorylases,* etc. The systematic name of *acetate kinase* (trivial name) for example, which catalyzes the following reaction is ATP— acetatephosphotransferase.

$$\text{ATP} + CH_3COOH \rightleftharpoons \text{ADP} + CH_3\overset{\overset{\displaystyle O}{\|}}{C}-OPO_3H_2$$

Creatine phosphoryl transferase, an important enzyme in muscle, catalyzes the transfer of the "energy-rich" phosphate group from creatine phosphate (CP) to adenosine diphosphate (ADP) to form adenosine triphosphate (ATP).

$$\underset{\text{(creatine phosphate)}}{\text{CP}} + \text{ADP} \xrightarrow[\textit{transferase}]{\textit{Creatine phosphoryl}} \underset{\text{(creatine)}}{\text{C}} + \text{ATP}$$

The so-called transaminases mediate the transfer of the amino group of an amino acid to an acid having a ketone group.

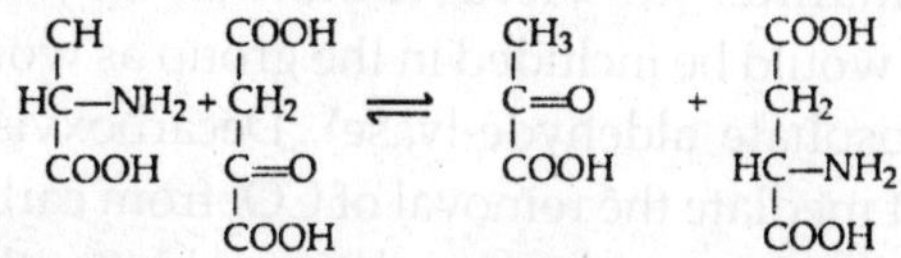

Alanine (amino acid) Oxaloacetic acid Pyruvic acid Aspartic acid

Kinases mediate the transfer of a phosphate group specifically from the ATP to particular substrates. The latter are thus converted to the corresponding phosphate esters, whereas the ATP is reduced to ADP. For example, the metabolism of glucose by most cells involves first its phosphorylation by the transfer of a phosphate group from ATP, a reaction which takes place only in the presence of a particular enzyme, *hexokinase.*

Hydrolases : are the enzymes that perform as their primary function the *hydrolysis* of a variety of compounds by water. Acetylcholinesterase which catalyses the cleavage of acetylcholine to choline and acetic acid, may be used as an example. This reaction takes place in the transmission of nerve impulses.

$$\underset{\text{Acetylcholine}}{CH_3CO-O-CH_2CH_2CH_2N^+(CH_3)_3} \underset{-H_2O}{\overset{+H_2O}{\rightleftharpoons}} \underset{\text{Acetic acid}}{CH_3COOH} + \underset{\text{Choline}}{HOCH_2CH_2N^+(CH_3)_3}$$

Hydrolases comprise a long list of enzymes named on the pattern of "Substrate hydrolases". Thus a lipase (trivial name) would be considered correctly as "glycerol ester hydrolase".

$$\text{Triglyceride} + H_2O \xrightarrow{\text{lipase}} \text{glycerol} + \text{fatty acids}$$

Other well known enzymes in this group are *phosphatases*, *peptidases*, and *amidases* etc.

Lyases : These are a group of enzymes that reversibly catalyze the removal of groups from substrates non-hydrolytically. Thus, fumarase (systematic name l-malate hydrolase) catalyzes the removal of water from malate in a reversible manner to yield fumarate. A *decarboxylase* (carboxylase would be included in the group as would aldolase (ketose-1-phosphate aldehyde-lyase). Decarboxylases are the enzymes that mediate the removal of CO_2 from carboxylic acid. For example, *pyruvic acid decarboxylase* accelerates the following reaction.

$$\underset{\text{Pyruvic acid}}{CH_3COCOOH} \xrightarrow{\text{lipase}} \underset{\text{Acetaldehyde}}{CH_3CHO} + CO_2$$

Isomerases or Mutases : These are the enzymes that catalyze the interconversion of a compound to one of its isomers. For example, in the anaerobic breakdown of carbohydrate to lactic acid, *triose phosphate isomerase* converts 3-phosphoglyceraldehyde to dihydroxyacetone phosphate.

Ligases or Synthetases : These are the enzymes that catalyze the linking together of two separate molecules, coupled with the breaking of a pyrophosphate bond. A triphosphate nucleotide, such as ATP presumably participates in the reaction.

$$\text{Thus, } X + Y + ATP \rightleftharpoons X\text{-}Y + AMP + P\text{-}P \text{ (Pyrophosphate)}$$

The systematic name of the enzyme catalyzing the above reaction is X : Y ligase (AMP). An excellent example of such a ligase is acetylcoenzyme A(CoA) synthetase.

$$\text{acetate} + \text{CoA-SH} + \text{ATP} \rightleftharpoons \text{acetyl CoA} + \text{AMP} + \text{P-P}$$

This enzyme is usually called *acetic thiokinase* but the systematic name would be acetate : CoA-SH-ligase (AMP).

Theories of Enzyme Action

According to the modern *collision theory* of chemical reactions, a catalyst increases the rate of a chemical reaction by participating in the formation of an activated and unstable complex of a lower energy state. Thus, in the presence of a catalyst, the required *energy of activation* is less, which means that there is now a lower energy barrier for the substrate molecules to overcome in order to undergo chemical reaction (or a change). A catalyst does this by interacting with one or more reactions in such a way that less energy is required to achieve the necessary bond reorganizations associated with the reaction.

The enzyme (E) as a biological catalyst performs this action by combining with the substrate molecule (S) to form a so-called *enzyme-substrate complex* (E-S). During the very brief existence of this complex, the enzyme activates the substrate for further reaction (E-Sa) and the end product (P) soon starts to form and finally dissociates from the enzyme, making the latter available for reacting with more substrate molecules. This process, as shown below, can be repeated several times:

$$\text{E} + \text{S} \rightleftharpoons \text{E-S} \rightleftharpoons \text{E-Sa} \rightleftharpoons \text{E-P} \rightleftharpoons \text{E} + \text{P}$$

In the above reaction E represents the enzyme, S the substrate, E-S enzyme-substrate complex, E-Sa enzyme-activated substrate complex, E-P enzyme-end product complex, and P the end product. These events are more conveniently described by the equation.

$$\text{E} + \text{S} \underset{k_2}{\overset{k_1}{\rightleftharpoons}} \text{ES} \xrightarrow{k_3} \text{E} + \text{P}$$

The theory thus assumes that the enzyme (E) combines with the substrate (S) to form a compound (ES) by a reversible reaction where k_1 is the rate constant for the formation of ES, and k_2 is the rate constant for the dissociation of ES to E and S. After the formation of ES, Substrate (S) is converted into the products, thus making enzyme (E) available for further combination with more substrate. The rate of conversion of ES to the products of the reaction may be indicated by the constant k_3.

Each enzyme-catalyzed reaction has a characteristic Km value, which is the Michaelis-Menten constant. This value is a measure of the tendency of the enzyme and the substrate to combine with each other.

$$K_m = \frac{k_2 + k_3}{k_1} = \frac{[E]\,[S]}{[ES]}$$

In this way the Km value is an index of the affinity of the enzyme for its particular substrate. It should be noted that *"greater the affinity of an enzyme for its substrate, the lower the Km value"*. This is because the Km value is numerically equal to the substrate concentration at which half of the enzyme molecules are associated with substrate (i.e., in the ES form).

Lock-and-key Theory of Enzyme Action : Each enzyme has a unique shape into which a complementary substrate fits quite easily just like a key fits into its lock. This is the so-called *lock-and-key theory* of enzyme action. The substrate binds to the enzyme with great precision. This binding involves atleast three points of contact with the enzyme.

Thus, enzyme performs its action by combining with some particular part of the substrate molecule (fig.). In other words, the substrate does not take up just any position on the enzyme molecule, but rather selects some small segment of the enzyme. These sites on the enzyme molecule that act as *substrate binders* or *activators*, or both are called *active sites*. The active site of an enzyme is formed by a number of *amino acid residues* whose side chains have two important roles : (1) they serve to *attract* and *orient* the substrate in a specific manner within the site (such amino acids are called *contact residues* and contribute in large degree to substrate specificity); and (2) they participate in the *formation of temporary bonds* with the substrate molecule. These bonds polarize the substrate, introduce strain into certain of its bonds and trigger the catalytic change (such amino acids are termed *catalytic residues).*

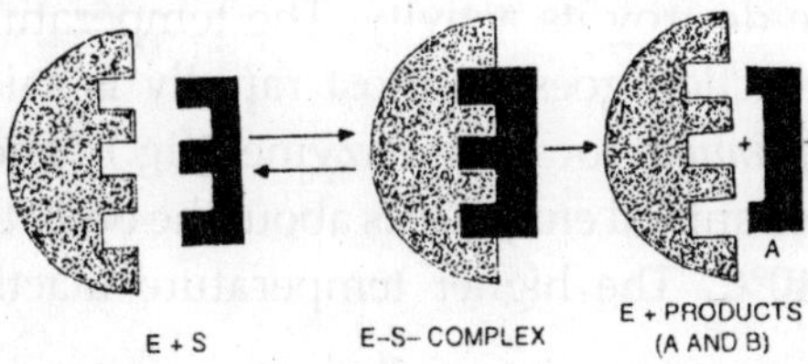

The formation of an enzyme-substrate complex illustrating the "lock and key" relationship between the substrate and active sites on the enzyme.

What happens after the formation of the enzyme-substrate-complex, depends upon the nature of enzyme, substrate and other factors. In some cases there is a transfer of electrons from the substrate to the enzyme (E-S complex), or in other cases the enzyme simply brings a substrate-molecule and a water-molecule in closer association so that the hydrolysis may occur.

Induced Fit Theory of Enzyme Action : According to this theory; first suggested as a general mechanism of enzyme action by D. *Koshland* (1963), enzyme changes its conformation when it combines with substrate. The theory proposes that the active site of the enzyme does not initially exist in a shape that is complementary to the substrate, but is *induced* to assume the complementary shape as the substrate binds. Thus, according to the induced fit model, the enzyme (or its active site) is *flexible.*

The energy required to bring about conformational changes in the enzyme and strain in the substrate comes form the *energy of binding*. The energy of binding, being maximized after a change in the conformation of the enzyme and substrate, might be primarily responsible for the greater increase in the rate of reaction of the correct substrate. Some recent studies of *W.J. Ray Jr.* provide striking evidence for the reduction of activation energy barriers by binding of a substrate *(Loewy et.al*, 1991).

Factors Influencing the Enzyme Activity : Many factors influence the activity of enzymes and those that alter the protein of the enzyme destroy its activity. The temperature at which the enzyme reaction goes on most rapidly is said to be the *temperature optimum* for that enzyme (fig.). The optimum temperature for animal enzymes is about the body temperature *i.e.*, 37°C to 40°C. The higher temperature inactivates most enzymes.

The pH of the medium (fig.) also influences the enzyme action, because each enzyme usually works best within a certain range of acidity or alkalinity. For example , *pepsin* of the gastric juice is most active at about pH 1.8, *trypsin* of the pancreatic juice at about pH 8.2. Thus, the *pH optimum* is characteristic for each enzyme and many have pH optima in neutral or slightly alkaline solutions. Excessive acidity or alkalinity causes destruction or *denaturation* of the enzyme protein, just as the high temperature causes heat denaturation.

The enzyme activity also depends upon the amount of substrate (fig.), because an enzyme will do its maximum work when there is enough substrate to combine with all the active sites of the enzyme molecule. In such a case no further increase in the substrate can increase the amount of reaction, for all the enzyme is being used.

Enzymes can be destroyed or their action can be *inhibited* by the effect of inhibitors like silver nitrate, copper sulphate, etc. The end products of the reaction also influence the rate of enzyme action. If they are allowed to accumulate, they will inhibit the activity of enzymes (feedback inhibition). Enzymes placed in water without a substrate lose their catalytic power rapidly, because they themselves are hydrolysed.

Effect of Hormones on the Enzyme Activity : In some cases there exists a close relationship between the enzymes and hormones. Hormones influence the enzyme activity in several ways. For instance, the balance between the sugar of the blood and the liver glycogen is influenced by the action of the *diabetogenic hormone* of the pituitary gland. This hormone tends to inhibit the action of the enzyme *hexokinase* which promotes the storage of sugar as glycogen. If the diabetogenic hormone is secreted in excess, sugar will not be stored in the liver as glycogen but will remain in the blood causing a higher level of the same.

However, the diabetogenic hormone is itself controlled by insulin. But if insulin is deficient, the diabetogenic hormone is free to inhibit the action of hexokinase. Thus, diabetes may be caused by an underproduction of the hormone insulin, or an overproduction of the diabetogenic hormone. Some hormones influence the digestive glands to produce their juices or secretions. They are discussed in the chapter on digestion. In this way, many enzymatic activities of our body depend more or less on hormones. Hormones may affect an enzyme activity as inhibitors or activators.

Industrial Enzymes and Enzyme Technology : Enzyme preparations, manufactured industrially—by separation of the enzyme system from its source , are known as the *industrial enzymes.* They are obtained from three main sources.

(i) *Plants* : Enzymes obtained from the plants include malt diastase, papain, uromelain, ficin, etc.

(ii) *Animals* : Important enzymes obtained from the animal tissues are pancreatic enzymes, pepsin, lipase, catalase, renin, etc.

(iii) *Microbes* : Cells of micro-organisms are used directly as crude enzyme preparations, or they may be used as a source of self-reproducing enzyme supply. An example of the first type is dried baker's yeast which does not reproduce or rarely reproduces during its use in the household. Example of the second type is every microbial inoculum used in a microbial process involving cell reproduction. The other examples of microbial industrial enzymes are amylase, protease, pectinase, invertase, and glucose oxidase, etc.

From fermentation methods it is now possible to obtain a large number of enzymes through micro-organisms and also to develop new systems which are not commercially available from animal or plant sources. Bacteria, fungi and yeasts are employed as the enzyme sources. All the processes for the manufacture of industrial enzymes belong either to:

(i) production in semi-solid culture or,

(ii) production by submerged fermentation.

While the former process has traditionally been used for the production of amylases and proteases, the latter is currently more in practice for the production of bacterial amylase and protease by *Bacillus subtilis*.

Immobilized Enzymes

Till recently enzymes were used in dilute aqueous media and it was rather difficult to recover such enzymes at the end of catalytic process.

However, the recovery of an enzyme is essential because its isolation, purification and crystallization is a difficult and costly process. Now this problem has been solved by attaching enzymes on a solid support material. Such attachment immobilizes the enzyme molecule and renders it insoluble in aqueous media.

Thus, the enzyme can be reused. The application of immobilized enzymes in medicine and industry, etc. is quite impressive. Some examples are the use of pepsin and renin in cheese making, the use of catalase and trypsin in increasing shelf life of milk, and application of hespiridinase in production of artificial sweetness.

Lysozyme

Lysozyme is an enzyme found in tears and saliva that can bring about the rupture of bacteria by hydrolyzing a specific linkage in the polysaccharide chains of bacterial cell walls. The lysozyme molecule is composed of a single chain of 129 amino acids linked in four places by disulfide bonds. Three-dimensional structure of lysozyme shows that the helical content of lysozyme is less than one-half of the 75% observed in myoglobin.

The molecule also contains a structure, "the antiparallel pleated sheet", which *Pauling* and *Corey* predicted to occur in certain fibrous proteins. One more interesting feature of lysozyme molecule is that the first 40 residues from the amino-terminal end form a compact helical structure. This could act as a "substructure" around which the rest of the molecule is folded as it is being synthesized on the ribosome.

Running down the middle of the molecule there is a *cleft,* which represents the binding site for the polysaccharide chain which is the enzyme's normal substrate. *Phillips* (1966) has suggested a specific mechanism for enzyme action of lysozyme. This mechanism provides the first direct confirmation of the induced fit theory of *Koshland* (1963).

Practical Application of Enzymes

Enzymes are widely used almost in every field where organic products of animal and plant origin are processed into consumer goods. Some of the major areas involving practical application of enzymes are as follows:

Medical Uses : A large number of enzymes are used in medical industry for diagnostic and therapeutic applications. For example, *glucose oxidase* is used in assay of glucose in body fluids; *proteases* are used for removing necrotic tissues, thereby enhancing wound healing; *asparagenase* is used for removing the essential amino acids from the blood, which eventually causes susceptible tumor cells to die. This possibility is being explored for leukemia therapy. *Urease* is used in clinical tests for measuring urea in blood.

Production of Foods and Food Ingredients : A good number of enzymes are used in the production of foods and food ingredients . For example, *bromelain* is used in baking; *capalase* is used in cheese making. Other enzymes used in food industry are catalase, cellulase, ficin, protease, glucose oxidase, pectinase, pepsin, etc.

Production of Beverages : Many enzymes are used in the production of fruit juices, fruit drinks, carbonated beverages, beer, wine and distilled beverages. Some of the enzymes used in brewery are catalase, pectinase, pectinol, rhozyme, and maltase, etc.

Leather Industry : During preparation of leather, enzymes like catalase, protease, and papain, etc. are used.

Paper and Textile Industry : Rhozyme is used in paper and textile industry and in photographic products; α-Amylase is used in the treatment of waste from paper manufacture.

Detergent Industry : Enzyme washing powders manufactured by incorporating proteases in presoak and heavy-duty washing powders remove protein from clothes having spots of blood, milk and egg yolk, etc., far more effectively than detergents alone. Amylases and lipases when incorporated into washing powders remove some stains quickly and easily. Dish washing powders containing amylase remove starch from crookeries.

Other Uses **:** In addition to the above, enzymes also find application in the manufacture of adhesives, in sewage disposal, animal feeding, tobacco processing, tea processing, sugar industry, pharmaceuticals and chemical and analytical reagents, etc.

The future of enzyme technology is bright. It is believed that if nitrogen-fixing enzymes could be harnessed in such a way that cereal crops could be grown with limited quantity of nitrogeneous fertilizer, and if economic conversion of cellulose into more useful compounds like glucose could be accomplished using enzymes, they will have a great impact on world economy.

6

The Coenzymes

In cellular physiology many enzymatic reactions are completed in the presence of coenzymes. These are compounds which function like the enzymes, *i.e.*, they speed up the biological reactions, but they are not proteins like the true enzymes.

***Definition :** A coenzyme may be defined as a particular kind of cofactor, i.e., a non-protein organic compound, or a carrier molecule functioning in conjunction with a particular enzyme.*

If the cofactor is firmly bound to the *apoenzyme* (the protein part of an enzyme), it is called a *prosthetic group* (*Gr. prosthesis*, in addition); and if, instead of being more or less permanently bound to the apoenzyme, the organic cofactor attaches itself to the enzyme protein only at the time of reaction, it is called a *coenzyme*.

In cellular processes sometimes hydrogen atoms or electrons are removed from one compound and transferred to another. In all such cases a specific enzyme catalyzes the removal, but a specific coenzyme must also be present to carry out the transfer. The coenzyme temporarily joins to, or accepts, the removed group of atoms and may subsequently hand over them to another acceptor compound.

Chemical Nature of Coenzymes

The majority of coenzymes are chemical derivatives of the *nucleotides* (nucleotide means a nitrogen base-pentose sugar-phosphate complex). More specifically, in most coenzymes the nitrogen base portion of the nucleotides is substituted by another chemical unit. This unit itself is usually a derivative of a particular vitamin. The following coenzymes are important in cellular physiology.

(i) Pyridine derivatives or Pyridine nucleotides (NAD and NADP).

(ii) Flavin derivatives or Flavin nucleotides (FMN and FAD).

(iii) Coenzyme Q.

(iv) Cytochromes.

(v) Coenzyme A.

(vi) Thiamine pyrophosphate (cocarboxylase).

Of these, the first four participate intimately with the enzymes of the respiratory chain, hence they are also called *respiratory coenzymes.*

Pyridine Nucleotides

Pyridine nucleotides, NAD and NADP, are derivatives of adenosine monophosphate (AMP), a typical nucleotide, and they are referred to as coenzyme I and coenzyme II respectively. The NAD in animal tissues is 0.5 to 3 mm, several times higher than the NADP, which ranges from 0.01 to 0.1 mm. In liver, however, the NADP is about one-third of NAD.

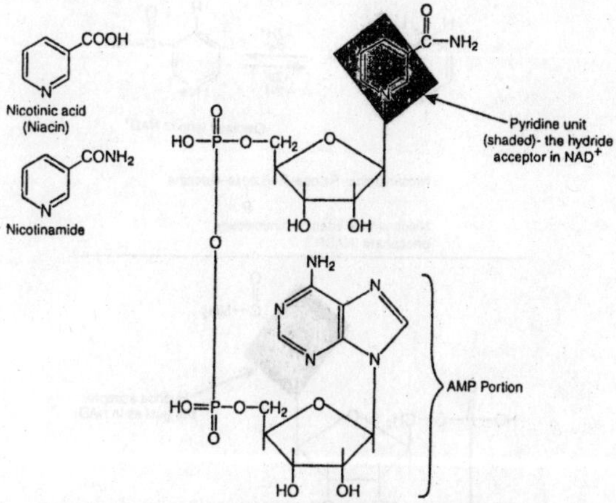

Nicotinamide-Ribose-P-P-Ribose-Adenine
Nicotinamide adenine dinucleotide (NAD^+)

The chemical structure of NAD.

Coenzyme I was formerly called *diphosphopyridine nucleotide* (DPN), but it is now more commonly known as *nicotinamide-adenine-dinucleotide* (NAD). The coenzyme II was similarly called *triphosphopyridine nucleotide* (TPN), but its more common name today is *nicotinamide-adenine-dinucleotide-phosphate* (NADP). The old names (DPN and TPN), originally proposed by *Warburg* in 1935, are now considered objectionable because in any of them a "phospho" group is not attached to a pyridine ring.

Nicotinamide Adenine Dinucleotide (NAD)

Structure : NAD is a pyridine nucleotide (Fig.). It consists of two nucleotides joined together at the phosphate groups (pyrophosphate bond). One nucleotide has adenine as its side chain, while the other has *nicotinamide* (a derivative of a vitamin B, *niacin* or *nicotinic* acid). A molecule of niacin possesses a so-called *pyridine* ring, hence the coenzyme forms of the vitamin are called *pyridine nucleotide coenzymes.* It is the pyridine unit of the molecule that serves specifically as the carrier of hydrogen atoms, as shown below:

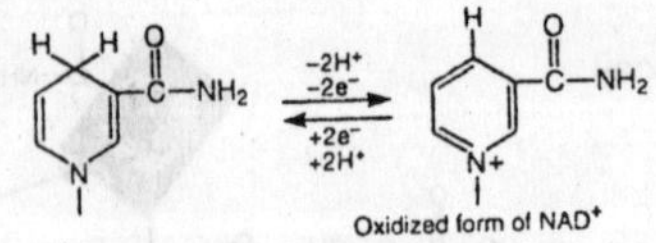

Nicotinamide–Ribose–P–Ribose–Adenine
P
Nicotinamide adenine dinucleotide phosphate ($NADP^+$)

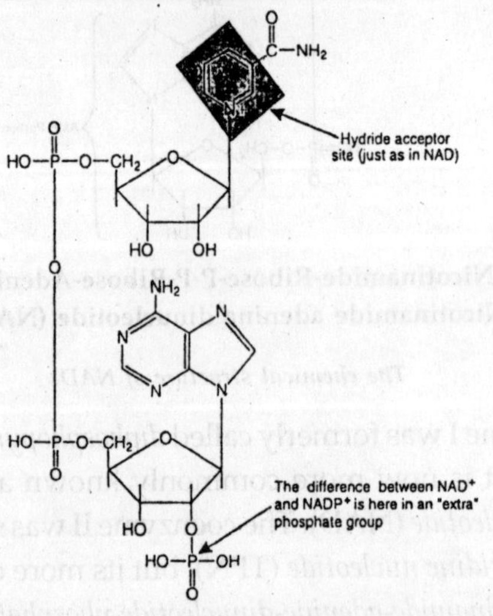

The chemical Structure of NADP.

Function: NAD functions in conjunction with the enzymes called *dehydrogenases*, the enzymes which catalyze the oxidation-reduction reactions. NAD is the coenzyme used in most reactions in which the free energy of substrate oxidation is conserved for subsequent ATP synthesis and thus, it functions in five of the six dehydrogenations in the oxidation of glucose. The following equation indicates how NAD serves as hydrogen-carrier or oxidizing agent:

$$MH_2 + NAD^+ \xrightarrow{dehydrogenase} M: + H^+ + NADH$$

where MH^2 represents any substrate or metabolite that loses the elements of hydrogen (H^- : and H^+), NAD^+ is the symbol for oxidized form of NAD, M : represents the oxidized form of the substrate after it has lost the elements of hydrogen and NADH is the symbol for the reduced form of NAD.

Nicotinamide Adenine Dinucleotide Phosphate (NADP)

Structure : NADP is a close relative of NAD. It also consists of two nucleotides joined together at the phosphate groups. One nucleotide has adenine as its side chain, while the other has nicotinamide. NADP has an extra phosphate group attached to the ribose of AMP (adenosine monophosphate) portion (Fig.). As in NAD, the pyridine unit of NADP serves as the carrier of hydrogen atoms.

Function : NADP also functions in the same way as NAD.

$$NADP^{+} + MH_2 \longrightarrow M: + H^{+} + NADPH$$

In this reaction $NADP^{+}$ is the symbol for oxidized form of NADP, and NADPH represents the reduced form of NADP. NADP is employed in processes by which reducing power is utilized for synthesis of a cell metabolite or for fatty acid synthesis . In both plants and animals, NADP is utilized in reactions for synthesis of steroids and many amino acids.

Role of NAD and NADP in Krebs Cycle : Here it may be mentioned that when hydrogen is removed from different substrates of the Krebs cycle, the hydrogen acceptors are NAD and NADP. From these coenzymes the hydrogen atoms and their electrons are passed on to the flavin nucleotides (FMN and FAD), cytochromes and finally to oxygen. For example, when a molecule of malic acid, which is one of the substrates of the Krebs cycle, is oxidized in the mitochondria, the following reaction takes place.

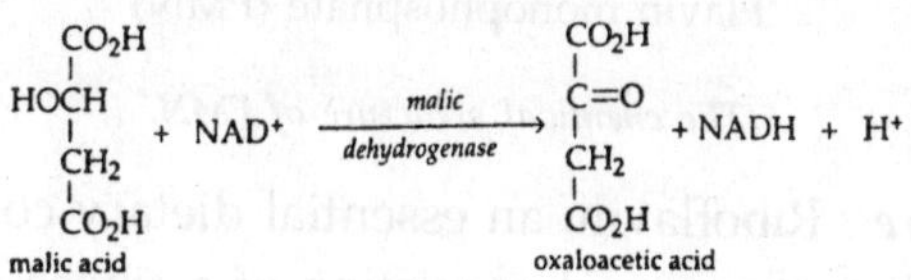

malic acid oxaloacetic acid

Thus, in the presence of an appropriate dehydrogenase two hydrogen atoms and electrons are removed from the substrate. In turn the oxidised pyridine nucleotide accepts two electrons and one proton in becoming reduced, and the other hydrogen is released as a proton. The NADH formed in the above reaction is in turn reoxidized by a flavoprotein of the respiratory chain. It should be noted that each dehydrogenase is usually highly specific for either NAD or NADP. In general, enzymes responsible for oxidations supplying energy to an organism utilize NAD, whereas those providing the energy for reductive synthesis utilize NADP (*Smith* et. al., 1983).

Flavin Nucleotides or Flavoproteins

A large group of respiratory enzymes use as their cofactor one of the two derivatives of *riboflavin* (vitamin B_2). They are *flavin mononucleotide* (FMN) and *flavin adenine dinucleotide* (FAD).

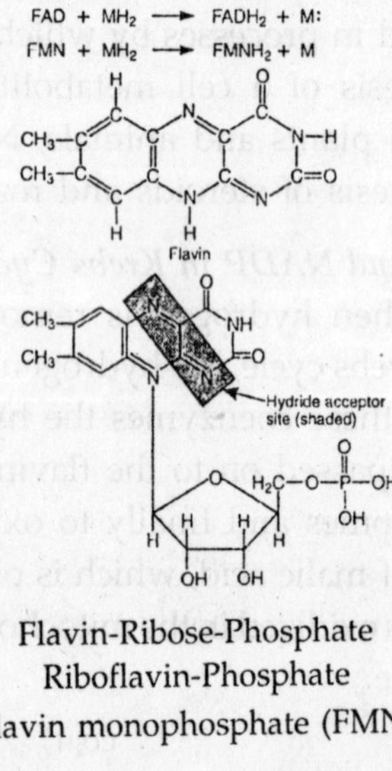

Flavin-Ribose-Phosphate
Riboflavin-Phosphate
Flavin monophosphate (FMN)

The chemical structure of FMN.

Structure : Riboflavin, an essential dietary constituent for mammals, is a compound consisting of a ribose portion, and a flavin portion, the latter being a complex triple ring structure. In cells, a phosphate group is linked to riboflavin resulting in a nucleotide-like complex known as *flavin mononucleotide* (FMN) or *riboflavin monophosphate* (Fig.). If FMN joins to AMP, a dinucleotide known as flavin adenine dinucleotide (FAD) is formed (Fig.).

Function : The combination of either FMN or FAD with an apoenzyme is called *flavoprotein* (FP). Flavoproteins catalyze the removal of hydride ion (H^-) and hydrogen ion (H^+) from a metabolite. In these coenzymes, it is the flavin portion of the molecule that provides the specific place for temporary attachment of hydrogen.

$$FAD + MH_2 \longrightarrow FADH_2 + M:$$

$$FMN + MH_2 \longrightarrow FMNH_2 + M:$$

In this reaction MH_2 represents a substrate, $FADH_2$ is the reduced form of FAD, and $FMNH_2$ is the reduced form of FMN.

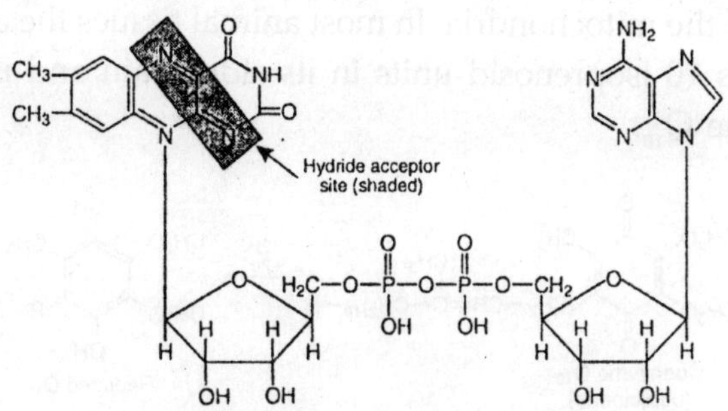

Flavin-Ribose-P-P-Ribose-Adenine
Flavin adenine dinucleotide (FAD)

The chemical structure of FAD.

An important source of hydrogen for this reaction is the reduced pyridine nucleotide.

$$H^+ + NADH + FAD \longrightarrow NAD^+ + FADH_2$$

However, in the case of the enzyme *succinate dehydrogenase*, which catalyzes the oxidation of succinic acid to fumaric acid, the FAD which is firmly joined to the enzyme is reduced and a pyridine nucleotide is not involved.

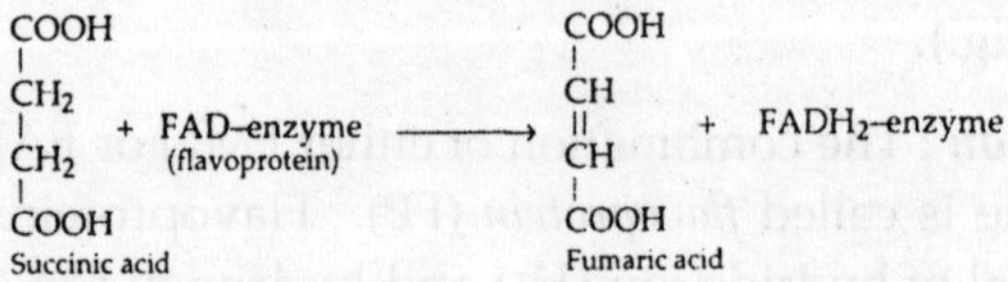

In all the cases reduced flavoproteins pass on their electrons to the cytochromes.

Coenzyme Q

This coenzyme is a quinone, known as ubiquinone, and is found mainly in the mitochondria but also in cell nuclei and microsomes, etc.

Structure : The coenzyme Q or ubiquinone (Fig.), consists of a quinone with a side chain whose length varies with the source of the mitochondria. In most animal tissues the quinone possesses 10 isoprenosid units in its side chain and is called coenzyme Q_{10}.

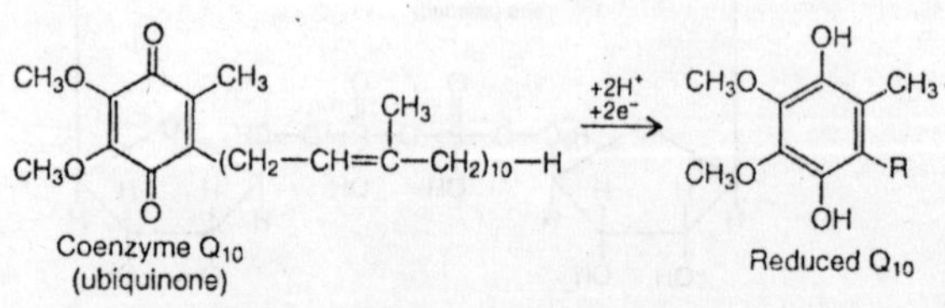

The Chemical structure of Coenzyme Q_{10}.

Function : The coenzyme Q is a necessary component of the electron transport chain in the mitochondria. It serves as an additional hydrogen carrier between the flavin coenzymes (FAD and FMN) and the cytochromes.

$$Q + FADH_2 \longrightarrow QH_2 + FAD$$

In the above reaction QH_2 represents the reduced form of Q. Reduced ubiquinone (QH_2) transfers its electrons to cytochrome *b* in the mitochondria.

Cytochromes

Cytochromes are found in all aerobic organisms and their amount varies according to the respiratory activity of the tissue. Thus, heart muscle is rich in cytochromes; but liver, kidney and brain have lesser amounts. The cytochromes are distinguished from one another by their absorption spectra.

Cytochromes (Gk. *kyto*, cell and *chroma*, pigment) form the last components of the electron transport chain. According to *Keilin* (1927), there are atleast 3 cytochromes of the *a*, *b* and c types in the mitochondria of every cell. In addition, cytochrome c_1 is also found. The available evidence indicates that in the intact mitochondria, the cytochromes react in sequence *i.e.*, from reduced coenzyme Q the electrons pass successively to b, c_1, c and a cytochromes. Finally the electrons are transferred from the reduced cytochrome a_3 or *cytochrome oxidase* to oxygen.

Structure : Cytochromes are conjugated proteins (haemoproteins) having an iron porphyrin as a prosthetic group. As their name (cell pigments) implies, they are coloured and the molecular unit responsible for the colour is the *porphyrin* skeleton made of four pyrrole units linked by —CH— bridges.

Function : As indicated above, the cytochromes accept electrons from the reduced coenzyme Q (QH_2) and are in turn alternately reduced and oxidized. The iron of the oxidised cytochrome is ferric iron and it is reduced to ferrous iron by the incorporation of an electron into the valence shell of the iron atom. Thus, one Fe^{3+} iron is able to accept one electron to become Fe^{2+}. Hence, if a cytochrome has to accept 2 electrons, there must be two Fe^{3+} ions or two molecules of cytochrome.

$$QH_2 + 2Fe^{3+} \longrightarrow Q + 2Fe^{2+} + 2H^+$$

Mitochondrial Cytochrome Complexes : In the main respiratory chain of mitochondria five principal fractions (complexes) that catalyze the mitochondrial electron transport chain, have been recognised (Fig.) and are :

Complex I : NADH $\xrightarrow{e}$ ubiquinone,

Complex II : Succinate $\xrightarrow{e}$ ubiquinone,

Complex III : dihydroubiquinone $\xrightarrow{e}$ ferricytochrome C

Complex IV : Ferrocytochrome C $\xrightarrow{e}$ O_2, and

Complex V : a Ca^{2+}-Mg^{2+}-dependent ATPase , is required for ATP synthesis; ADP + Pi $\rightarrow$ ATP

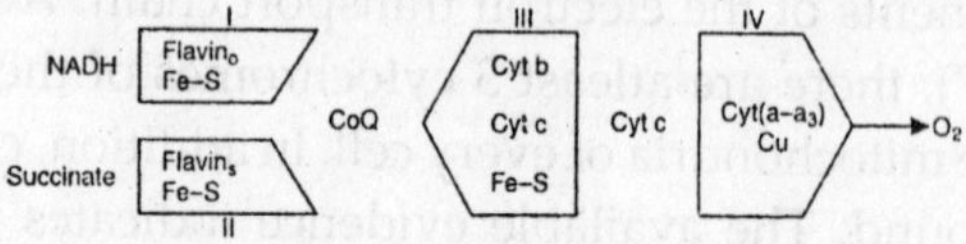

Mitochondrial cytochrome complexes of the respiratory chain.

Cytochrome b complexes : The b-type cytochromes are electron-carrier proteins with non-covalently bound heme (protoporphyrin IX Fe) as **a** functional group. About 80 per cent of cytochrome b is in complex III, the mitochondrial ubiquinol : cytochrome c reductase, and about 20 percent is in mitochondrial succinate reductase (Complex II). The cytochrome b of complex III is involved in the second site of phosphorylation of mitochondrial oxidative phosphorylation. The single structural gene for yeast cytochrome b contains about 900 base pairs and is composed of three exons, or coding regions, interrupted by two introns (non-coding regions) containing from 2000 to 4000 base pairs.

Cytochrome b_5 : It is tightly bound to membranes of the endoplasmic reticulum and is implicated in a number of NADPH-linked microsomal hydroxylation reactions including in hepatic microsomes in elongation of some fatty acids. Cytochrome b_5 is also found in erythrocytes and participates in reduction of methelglobin to haemoglobin and NADH-cytochrome b_5 reductase is its natural electron donor.

Cytochrome c : Mammalian cytochrome c is a globular electron-carrier protein of 104 residues (MW = 12,400) with a heme moiety (iron protoporphyrin IX) attached covalently by two thioether linkages to cysteniyl residues in the polypeptide chain. Unique among the mitochondrial cytochromes the iron of ferricytochrome c can be reduced or reoxidized. Ferrocytochrome c is dimagnetic and unlike ferrohaemoglobin, it does not combine with O_2 or CO, nor does it reoxidize in the presence of O_2. The cytochromes c act as components of the electron- transport chain of mitochondria, accepting electrons from cytochrome bc_1 complex and donating electrons to the cytochrome oxidase (aa3) complex. Cytochrome c mixed with phospholipids also serve as a substrate for cytochrome oxidase by providing binding site for anionic groups on cytochrome oxidase.

Cytochrome P_{450} : This class of cytochromes occur in most animal tissues, plants and micro-organisms, and catalyze the mono-oxygenation of a vast variety of hydrophobic substances. The liver P_{450} system catalyzes hydroxylation of aliphatic and aromatic carbons and is also involved in N-oxidation, sulfoxidation, epoxidation, N-, S- and O- dealkylation, peroxidation, deamination, desulfuration, dehalogenation and detoxification reactions. It acts on a vast array of substrates as normal metabolites, xenobiotic compounds, drugs, insecticides (as DDT) including many carcinogens. In addition, synthesis of many steroids also requires action of cytochrome P_{450}, specific for cholesterol side-chain cleavage.

Cytochrome a_3 : Cytochrome a_3 or *cytochrome oxidase* is synthesized jointly on mitochondrial and cytoplasmic ribosomes and it is one of the few enzymes capable of reducing molecular oxygen to water. Cytochrome oxidase from various sources contain seven sub-units. Reduced cytochrome a_3 has the ability to transfer electrons to molecular oxygen and thereby reduce the latter to water. Two molecules of reduced cytochrome a_3 are required to furnish the two electrons necessary for the reduction of one atom of oxygen, and two protons are required to balance the reaction :

$$2 \text{ cytochrome } a_3\text{-}(Fe^{2+})+2H^{+}+1/2O_2 \rightarrow 2 \text{ cytochrome } a^3\text{-}(Fe^{3+})+H_2O$$

Thus, the overall reaction catalyzed is :

$$4 \text{ cytochrome c -}(Fe^{2+}) + O_2 + 4H^{+} \rightarrow 4 \text{ cytochrome c }(Fe^{3+})+2H_2O$$

As cytochrome oxidase is the site of reduction of most cellular O_2, this mechanism (4-electron reduction of O_2 by cytochrome oxidase) ensures that the toxic, partially reduced intermediate forms of oxygen, such as O_2^- are not produced. Thus, cytochrome a_3 is the last hydrogen carrier of the respiratory chain and is referred to as the *terminal oxidase.*

Cytochromes a and a_3 also function in conserving the released energy for electron transfer for the formation of a proton gradient across the inner mitochondrial membrane required for ATP synthesis during oxidative phosphorylation.

Bacterial Cytochromes : The bacterial cell membrane contains dehydrogenases, cytochromes, and iron-sulfur centres that conduct oxidative phosphorylation. Bacterial cytochromes resemble in absorption spectra to cytochromes *a*, *b* and *c*, but differ a lot in their structural and functional properties from those of eukaryotes.

Coenzyme A

One of the coenzymes carrying not hydrogen but another specific group of atoms is coenzyme A (CoA). The discovery of coenzyme A by the American biochemist Dr. *Fritz Lipmann* earned him the Nobel Prize in 1955. The complete chemical synthesis of the coenzyme A was described by *Khorana* in 1959.

Structure : A molecule of coenzyme A consists of 3 parts: a phosphate derivative of ADP, a vitamin known as *pantothenic acid,* and a chain of nitrogen, carbon and sulphur atoms (Fig.). The pantothenic acid portion of the molecule is required in the mammalian diet and it also occurs in nature in combination with β-mercaptoethylamine as pantetheine. The latter is an intermediate in the pathway of CoA formation in mammalian liver and some micro-organisms. In short form, coenzyme A is written as CoA or CoASH. The SH refers to the sulphydryl group of coenzyme A.

Function : Coenzyme A serves as the carrier of a molecular group called *acetyl.* The latter becomes attached to the sulphur end of CoA and acetyl coenzyme A is formed (Fig.).

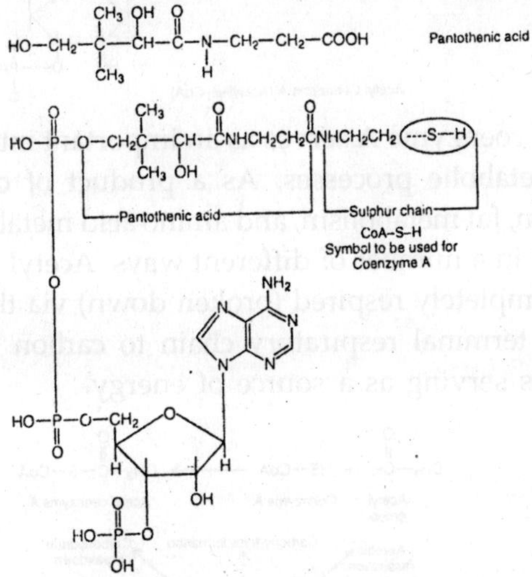

The chemical structure of pantothenic acid and coenzyme A.

Like the —O ~ P— bond which is found in the high-energy phosphates, the —S ~ C— bond too is a high-energy bond. Thus, coenzyme A serves both as *acetyl carrier* and an *energy carrier*. It is an important carrier in the respiratory transformation of pyruvic acid to acetyl coenzyme A.

$$\underset{\text{pyruvic acid}}{CH_3COCOOH} + CoASH \longrightarrow \underset{\text{acetyl CoA}}{CH_3COSCoA} + CO_2 + H_2$$

Acetyl Coenzyme A

The acetyl coenzyme A or "active acetyl" was discovered by *Lynen*. It is an energy-rich compound (thioester) whose Δ F′ of hydrolysis is —8000 cal/mole.

$$CH_3COSCOA + H_2O \longrightarrow CH_3COO + CoASH + H^+$$

acetyl CoA coenzyme A

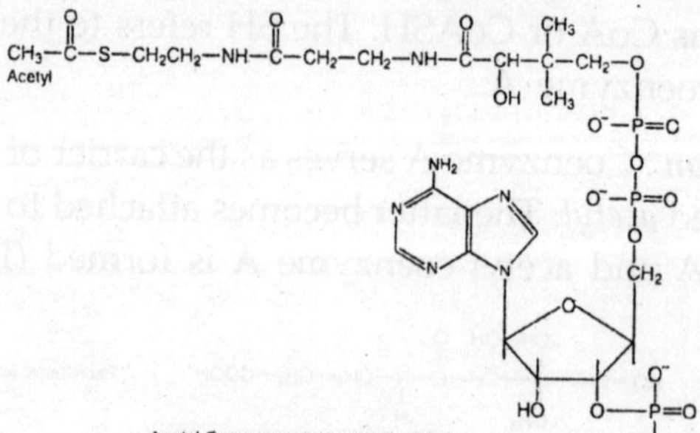

Acetyl Coenzyme A (Acetyl–S–CoA)

Acetyl coenzyme A serves as an important intermediate in several metabolic processes. As a product of carbohydrate metabolism, fat metabolism, and amino acid metabolism, it can be utilized in a number of different ways. Acetyl coenzyme A may be completely respired (broken down) via the citric acid cycle and terminal respiratory chain to carbon dioxide and water, thus serving as a source of energy.

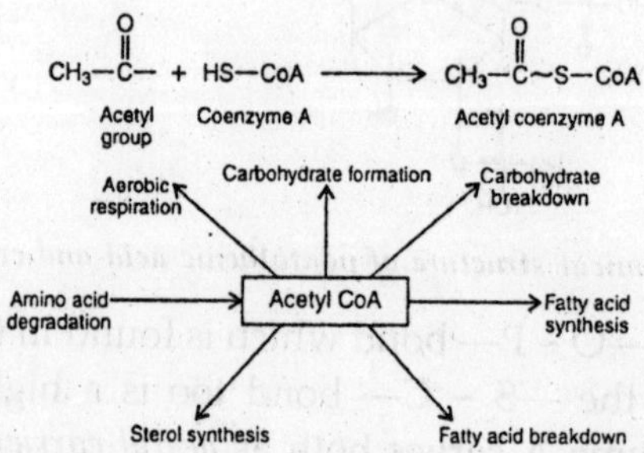

The chemical structure and the central role of acetyl coenzyme A in linking carbohydrate, lipid, and protein metabolism.

$$CH_3COSCoA + 3H_2O \rightarrow CoASH + 2CO_2 + 4H_2$$

The hydrogen atoms of the above reaction are passed on to the respiratory chain and the output is $4H_2O$ and 12 ATP.

Acetyl coenzyme A is also a building unit in fatty acid synthesis, carbohydrate synthesis and sterol synthesis. The important role of acetyl coenzyme A in linking carbohydrate, lipid and protein metabolism is shown in the (Fig.).

Thiamine Pyrophosphate

The removal of CO_2 from pyruvic acid requires a coenzyme called *thiamine pyrophosphate* (TPP) or cocarboxylase. It is a derivative of thiamine or vitamin B_1 (Fig.).

$$\underset{\text{Pyruvic acid}}{CH_3COCOOH} \xrightarrow[Mg^{2+}]{\textit{Cocarboxylase}} \underset{\text{acetaldehyde}}{CH_3CHO} + CO_2$$

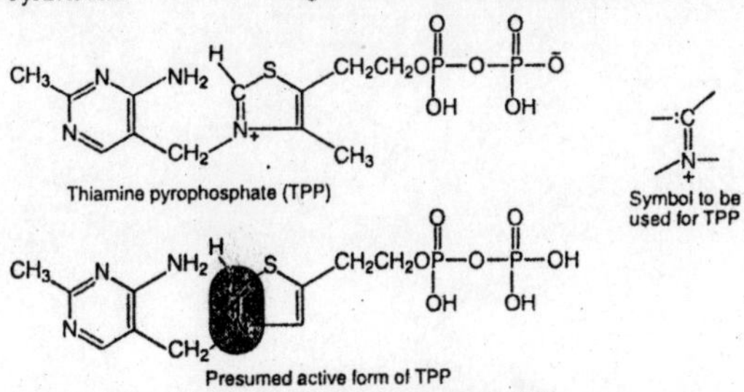

Fig. The chemical structure of TPP.

7

Excretion System

Excretion may be defined as the separation and elimination of the metabolic wastes from the body usually in an aqueous solution. The waste materials are of several kinds and vary not only from animal to animal, but also in the same animal from time to time. However, the term excretion is generally used with reference to the elimination of the *nitrogenus* waste products from the animal body.

During the oxidative metabolism of carbohydrates, *carbon dioxide* and *water* are formed as excretory products. The bile pigments *bilirubin* and *biliverdin* that are formed in the liver by the break down of haemoglobin are excretory substances which pass out through the intestine. The breakdown of proteins results in *amino acids,* the excess of which are excreted. While some aquatic animals excrete their extra nitrogen in the form of *amino acids* as such, most of the animals degrade their excess amino acids to *ammonia, uric acid* or *urea.*

Deamination : The first stage in the breakdown of amino acids is the removal of their nitrogenous groups as ammonia.

Removal of the amino groups (-NH_2) which converts the amino acid into a keto acid is called *deamination.* Such deamination results from the action of a variety of enzymes, which are either oxidative or hydrolytic.

Nature of Excretory Products

In vertebrates, deamination takes place particularly in liver cells, where any amino acid excess supplied by eaten food is deaminated. Ammonia produced in this way is highly toxic and must be disposed off. Elimination often occurs in the form of unchanged ammonia or in the form of a more complex nitrogenous substance which is either uric acid or urea. Based on the nature of the nitrogenous excretory end-product, animals are classified into 3 main categories :

(i) ammonotelic

(ii) uricotelic

(iii) ureotelic.

Ammanotelic Animals (Ammonotelism) : Animals which excrete their nitrogenous wastes as ammonia are said to be *ammanotelic.* Excretion of ammonia which is presumed to be the primitive excretory material, is especially suited to an aquatic habitat. Ammonia is highly soluble in water with which it form ammonium hydroxide (NH_4OH).

The latter passes readily across the cell membranes and is dispersed into the surrounding water. Ammonia is found as the chief excretory product in the majority of primitively aquatic animals, certain protozoa, spongs, polyehaete annelids, crustaceans, some molluscs and teleost fishes.

It is also excreted by secondarily aquatic animals such as the larvae of the insects *Aeschna* and aquatic tortoises and turtles. Anuran (amphibian) tabdpoles, excrete mainly ammonia, whereas the adults produce urea.

Ureotelic Animals (Ureotelism)

Animals which excrete their nitrogen predominantly in the form of uric acid are called *uricotelic.* All genuinely terrestrial animals, including insects, terrestrial gastropods, terrestrial reptiles (snakes, lizards) and birds excrete mainly uric acid. Insects and land snails excrete solid pellets of uric acid, whereas reptiles and birds void a thick paste of uric acid crystals.

Ureotelic Animals (Ureotelism) : Animals which excrete urea as their major excretory product are said to be *ureotelic.* Urea is a useful product for a semi-terrestrial animal that is not exposed to a scarcity of water, but is not necessarily surrounded by large quantities of it.

It is, therefore the main product of some earthworms, shore gastropods, adult amphibians and the semi-terrestrial tortoises and turtles. Elasmo-branch fishes and mammals are special cases that also excrete urea. In humans, the blood contains about .04 g/100 ml of urea, whereas the level of urea in the bladder is 2.0 g/100 ml of urine.

Although ammonia, uric acid and urea are the major excretory substances, there are a few more types of nitrogenous excretory products.

1. *Amino Acids :* Unio, linear and asterias.
2. *Trimethylamine Oxide :* Marine teleost fishes excrete a large proportion of their nitrogen-as trimethylamine oxide, a soluble non-toxic substance. It resembles in its properties with urea.
3. *Guanine :* Spiders excrete almost exclusively a substance guanine which resembles with uric acid. Guanine is even less soluble than uric acid and, therefore, requires no water for its elimination.
4. *Ornithinic Acid :* It is excreted in small amounts by

birds and is formed by a combination of benzoic acid in food with the amino acid ornithine.

5. *Creatine* : Mammals excrete creatine which is synthesized in the liver from three amino acids: arginine, glycine and methionine.
6. *Creatinine* : Mammals contain a small quantity of creatinine in their blood (1 mg/100 ml), which is a derivative of creatine. The excess is eliminated along with urine.

It should be remembered, however, that no animal excretes one type of product exclusively.

Functional Architecture of Mammalian Kidney : The kidney is a compound tubular gland, adapted to filtering wastes from the blood. It is enclosed in a strong capsule of connective tissue that contains a few smooth muscle fibres.

When cut open longitudinally, the kidney is seen to consist of an outer *cortex* and an inner *medulla;* they both contain the uriniferous tubules.

Cortex : The cortex is granular in appearance because the tubules here are much convoluted and it also contains the Malpighian corpuscles. The cortex overlies the bases of medullary pyramids and dips down between them. These displaced portions of cortex which invade the medullary theory and called the renal columns of Bertin. When viewed with a magnifying lens it becomes evident that the cortex is not uniform in texture. It is subdivided into alternating radial tracts known as rays and labyrinths. The rays are radially striate because they contain the straight parts of proximal tubules and the collecting ducts. They are continuous with the striate medulla, hence called "medullary rays", though cortical rays is an appropriate term for them. The labyrinths have a granular appearance because the convoluted tubules, which compose them, are cut irregularly. Among fresh tubules glomeruli may be seen as bright red points.

Medulla : The medulla looks striated as the tubules run through it in a straight course radiating towards the pelvis. The medulla consists of 10 to 15 conical masses, the renal pyramids, whose bases are adjacent to the cortex and whose apices form the papillae. Two or three pyramids commonly fuse and end in one common papilla. These papillae project into cup-shaped channels known as calyces. The spaces between calyces are part of the renal sinus and are filled with adipose tissue, vessels and nerves. The calyces join to form the pelvis which is the expanded beginning of the ureter. In the medulla are running in a straight course.

Hilum : The Mecial concave border of a kidney contains a notch known as the hilum through which the renal artery enters and renal vein and ureter leave the kidney.

Uriniferous Tubule

A complete uriniferous tubule consistes of two component parts :

(i) the secretory tubule or nephron which is long and unbranched.

(ii) the excretory portion which is branched, tree-like system of excretory ducts.

Secretory Tubule : It consists of the following parts :

(1) A dilated blind end, the glomerular (Bownan's) capsule, which is invaginated to enclose a tuft of convoluted blood capillaries, the glomerulus. The whole structure is called a Malpighian (renal) corpuscle.

(2) The tubule leaves the capsule by a constricted rock, passing into the greatly contorted proximal convoluted tubule.

The free surface of an epithelial cell lining the tubular lumen bears a prominent brush border for resorptive activities.

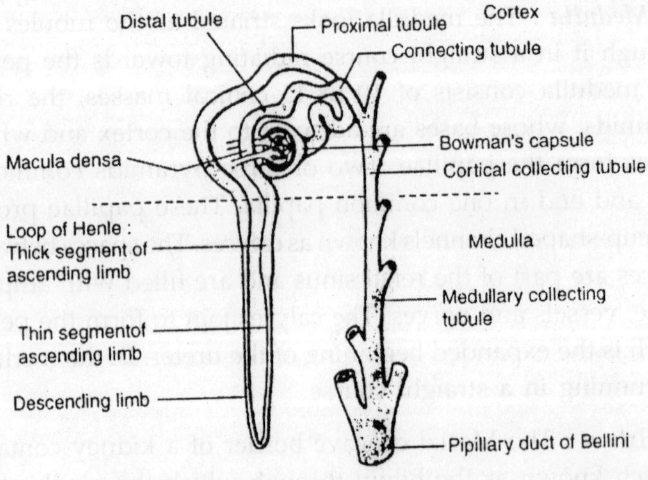

The Structure of a uniniferous tubule.

(3) The tubule then takes a straight course down to the medulla, where it doubles round and comes up again to the cortex. The loop thus formed is called the loop of Henle and is divided into three segments :

(a) *thinck descending segment* which is actually the straight portion of proximal convoluted tubule.

(b) *thin segment* which runs a direct, radial course in the medulla; it makes a sharp hair-pin bend and extends past the apex of Henle's loop.

(c) *thick ascending segment* of loop which is a straight radial tubule; there is an abrupt transition from the squamous epithelium of thin segment into cuboidal epithelium.

This is relatively impermeable to water and salts.

(4) The tubule leaves the medullary ray and enters the cortical tissue again, becoming the distal convoluted tubule, it lies near its own Malpighian corpuscle. This segment is short in comparison to the proximal convoluted tubule. It is narrower and less contorted.

The epithelium is cuboidal; there is a large lumen and an obvious brush border is lacking.

Excretory Portion

(5) The tubule then straightened out again, and by a short connecting tubule joins a straight, collecting tubule which passes down in a medullary ray, to enter a medullary pyramid.

On the way it receives other junctional tubules and forms a tree-like system.

(6) Finally, at large straight tubule, the papillary duct (of Bellini) opens into the pelvis at the apex of the papilla.

Regional Differences in Nephron Structure (Cortical and Juxtamedullary Nephrons) : Although each nephron has all the components described earlier, there are some differences, depending on how deep the nephrons lie within the kidney mass. Those nephrons that have glomeruli located in the outer cortex are called cortical nephrons; they have short loops of Henle that penetrate only a short distance into the medulla.

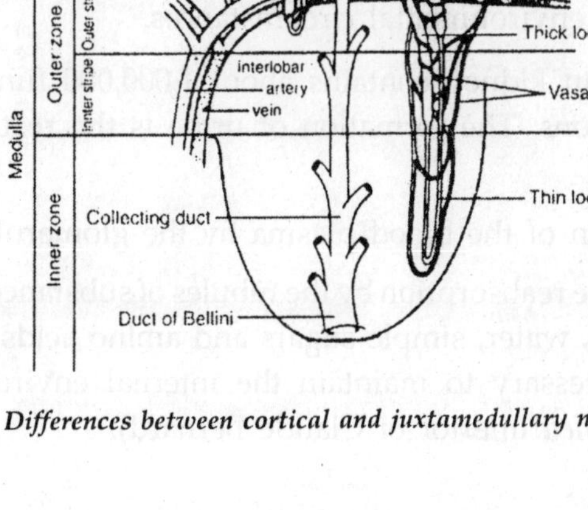

Differences between cortical and juxtamedullary nephrons

About 20 to 30 percent of the nephrons have glomeruli that lie deep in the renal cortex near the medulla and are called *Juxtamedullary nephrons.* These nephrons have long loops of Henle that dip deeply into medulla, in some cases all the way to tips of the renal papillae.

The vascular structures supplying the juxtamedullary nephrons also differ from those of the cortical nephrons. For the cortical nephrons, the entire tubular system is surrounded by an extensive network of peritubular capillaries. For the juxtamedullary nephrons, long efferent arterioles extend from the glomeruli down into the outer medulla and then divide into specialized peritubular capillaries called *vasa recta* that extend downward into the medulla, lying side by side, with the loops of Henle. Like the loops of Henle, the vasa recta return toward the cortex and empty into the cortical veins. This specialized network of capillaries in the medulla plays an essential role in the formation of a concentrated urine.

Formation of Urine

The kidney is the main secretory organ of the body and the fluid separated from plasma by its activity is the urine. In contrast to other secretions, however, urine exhibits a remarkable range of volume and composition. The kidney aids in regulating the volume and composition of body fluids by virtue of its ability to alter the nature of urine with varying metabolic and environmental circumstances.

Each human kidney contains about 1,000,000 functional units or nephrons. The formation of urine is the result of 3 process :

(1) filtration of the blood plasma by the glomeruli.

(2) selective reabsorption by the tubules of substances such as salts, water, simple sugars and amino acids which are necessary to maintain the internal environment (the *milieu* interior of Claude Bernard).

(3) secretion by the tubules of substances from the blood into the tubular lumen for excretion into the urine. This latter secretory process involves the handling of potassium, uric acid, organic anions and hydrogen ion. It serves, both as a means of regenerating components of the blood buffers and as a means of eliminating potentially harmful substances.

Filtration : The first step in urine formation is filtration of the blood plasma. A large volume of blood, approximately 1 litre/minute flows through the kidneys at rest. Filtration takes place through the semi-permeable walls of the glomerulus and the Bowman's capsule. The glomerulus is a tuft or knot of capillaries contained in the Bowmari's capsule. Each glomerulus receives blood from and *afferent* arteriole and discharges its blood into and *efferent arteriole*. Because the calibre of the efferent arteriole is smaller than that of the afferent arteriole., there develops a resistance to blood flow out of the glomeruli. As a result, a glomerular hydrostatic pressure (GHP) of about 60 mm Hg builds up in the glomerulus. This pressure is opposed by the blood colloidal osmotic pressure (BCOP), about 32 mm Hg, and by eapsular hydrostatic pressure (CHP) of about 18 mm Hg inside the Bowman's capsule.

$$60 - 32 - 18 = 10 \text{ mm Hg.}$$

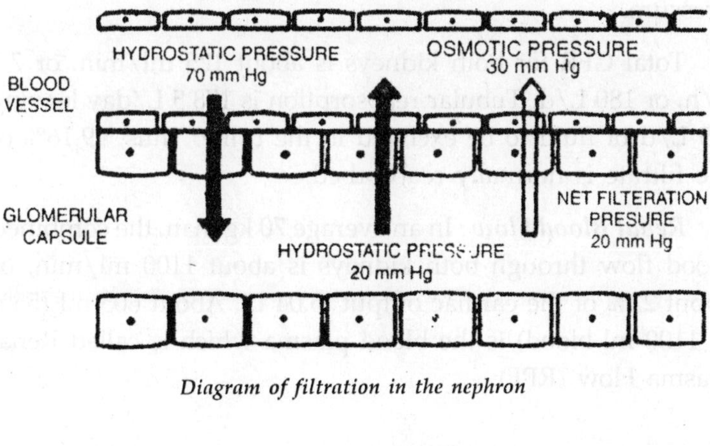

Diagram of filtration in the nephron

The molecular size of a substance present in the blood determines whether it is possible for it to pass through the filter substances of a low molecular weight filter from the blood into the Bowman's capsule due to effective filtration pressure (EFP). these include water, amino acids, salts fatty acids, glucose, urea, uric acid, creatinine and toxins etc,. The contents of the blood which are of high molecular weight, such as the red blood the glomerulus as they are unable to pass through this semi-permeable membrane.

The fluid thus produced is called the nephric or glomerular nitrate.

Glomerular Filtration Rate (GFR) equals the product of Glomerular Capillary Filtration Coefficient, K_f and the Net (Effective) Filtration pressure (EFP).

$$GFR = K_f \times \text{Net Filtration Pressure}$$

Glomerular Capillary Filtration Coefficient (K_f) is estimated by dividing the rate of GFR by Net Filtration Pressure.

$$K_f = GFR/\text{Net Filtration Pressure}$$

Since total GFR for both kidneys is about 125 ml/min. and the net filtration pressure is 10 mm Hg., the normal K_f is calculated to be about 12.5 ml/min./mm Hg of filtration pressure.

Total GFR for both kidneys is about 125 ml/min. or 7.5 L/h, or 180 L/d. Tubular reabsorption is 178.5 L/day leaving 1.5 L/d of fluid to be excreted in the urine. Thus, 99.16% of the filtrate is normally reabsorbed.

Renal Blood Flow : In an average 70 kg man, the combined blood flow through both kidneys is about 1100 ml/min, or about 22% of the cardiac output (5.04 L). About 605 ml (55% of 1100 ml blood) is the blood plasma which is called Renal Plasma Flow (RPF).

Filtration Fraction : The ratio of GFR (125 ml) to RPF (605 ml) is called Filtration fraction. It is 0.20

125/605 = 0.20.

5 L	=	5000 ml (C.O.) × 55% (Plasma)
	=	2750 ml

Out of this only 605 ml of plasma passes through kidneys,

$\therefore$ 605/2750 = 22%

The filtration fraction is calculated as follows :

Filtration Fraction = GFR/ RPF

125/605 = 0.2.

Selective Reabsorption

The glomerular filtrate contains many substances necessary for normal metabolism, such as water, glucose, amino acids, and electrolytes, as well as substances to be excreted and removed, such as urea, creatinine, and uric acid. Selective reabsorption is the process by which essential constituents of the glomerular filtrate are reabsorbed into the body, during its passage through the kidney tubules. It is also significant in the maintenance of fluid and electrolyte balance and the alkalinity of the blood (pH 7.4).

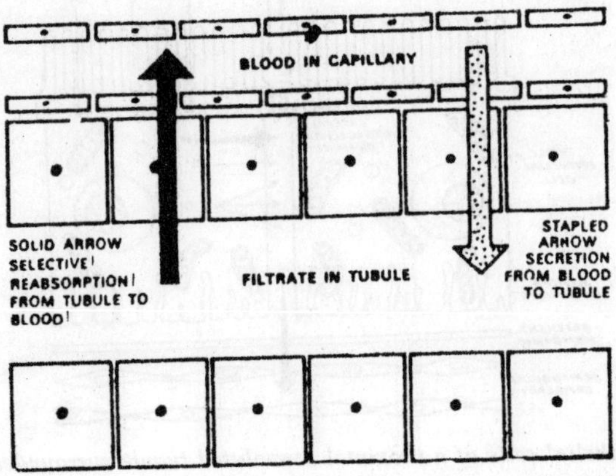

Diagram of selective reabsoption and secretion in the nephron.

The nephric filtrate collects within the Bowman's capsule and then passes into the proximal convoluted tubule. The cells of the proximal tubule have a well, developed brush border (microvilli) against the lumen, and the opposite side (against the peritubular blood capillaries) is packed with mitochondria. The microvilli greatly increase the surface area exposed to the nephric flltrater whereas mitochondria provide energy in the form of ATP for the active transport of some substances.

Inorganic compounds, when in solution become ionized. For example.

$$NaCl \rightleftharpoons Na^+ + Cl^-$$

Sodium chloride, glucose, amino acids and water first diffuse passively into the epithelial cell from the tubular lumen. *Sodium, glucose* and *amino acids* are then actively-transported (thick arrow) into the intercellular space (stippled area) *Chloride* moves passively by diffusion with the electrochemical gradient (due to potential difference). The materials reabsorbed by the proximal tubule are returned to the blood by peritubular capillaries. About 80% of the water in the nephric filtrate is reabsorbed by the proximal tubules. This fraction is referred to as the obligatory water reabsorption—a passive process.

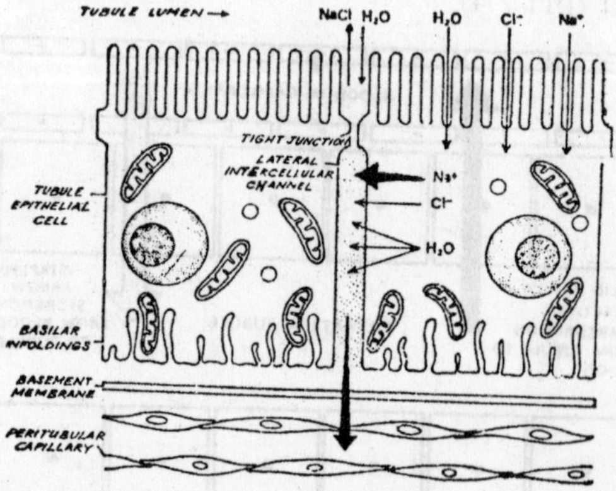

Epithelial cells of a proximal convoluted tubule surrounded by a peritubular blood capillary.

In the distal tubule, a more selective accurately regulated reabsorption of substances takes place. Here, more water (about 13%) is reabsorbed with the help of a pituitary hormone ADH which increases the permeability of the distal tubules to water. Distal tubular reabsorption is called the facultative water reabsorption—a process aided by the hormone.

In addition, the distal tubules help of preserve a constant pH in the blood (7.4) by exchanging hydrogen ions for sodium tends to rise. An adrenocortiosteriod aldosterone promotes the reabsorption of Na^+ in this case.

Tubular Secretion or Augmentation : It is a supporting mechanism which supplements the filtration-reabsorption mechanism. The cells of the tubules remove *non-threshold substances* and *foreign material* from the blood. They are actively transported into the tubular lumen against an electro-chemical gradient, i.e., to say they are secreted.

Examples of substances secreted by the tubular epithelium in man are *creatinine,* and *H^+ (ions);* certain drugs such as *pencillin* and *para aminohippuric acid (PAH).* NH_3 is excreted by passive diffusion.

Kidney Conserves Water by Excreting a Concentrated Urine : When there is a water deficit in the body, the kidney forms a concentrated urine by continuing to excrete solutes while increasing water reabsorption and decreasing the volume of urine formed. The human kidney can produce a maximal urine concentration of 1200 to 1400 mOsm/L, four to five times the osmolarity of plasma.

Some desert animals, such as the Australian hopping mouse, can concentrate urine to as high as 10,000 mOsm/L. This ability allows this mouse to survive in the desert without drinking water; sufficient water can be obtained through the food ingested and water produced in the body by metabolism of the food. On the other hand animals adapted to aquatic environments, such as the beaver, have minimal urine concentrating ability; they can concentrate the urine to only about 500 mOsm/L.

The basic requirements for forming a concentrated urine are (1) a high level of ADH, which increases the permeability of the distal tubules and collecting ducts to water, thereby allowing these tubular segments to avidly reabsorb water, and (2) a high osmolarity of the renal medullary interstitial fluid, which provides the osmotic gradient necessary for water resorption to occur in the presence of high levels of ADH. This process involves the operation of the countercurrent mechanism.

Countercurrent Mechanism of Urine Concentration : The kidneys produce concentrated urine by a complex sequence of events. The concentrating mechanism depends upon the maintenance of a gradient of increasing osmolarity along the medullary pyramids. This gradient exists because of the operation of the *loops of Henle* as Countercurrent Multipliers and the *vasa recta* as Countercurrent Exchanger.

A countercurrent system is a system in which the inflow runs parallel to, counter to, and in close proximity to the outflow for some distance, *e.g.*, the descending and ascending limbs of the loops of Henle.

Counter Current Multiplier System

1. The thick ascending limb on the loop of Henle actively transports Na^+ (Cl^-) by passive diffusion) out of the tubular lumen into the surrounding medullary interstitial tissue to establish a concentration gradient of 200 mOsm/L between the tubular fluid and the interstitial fluid.
2. The tubular fluid in the descending limb of the loop of Henle and the interstitial fluid quickly reach osmotic equilibrium because of osmosis of water out of the descending limb.

3. As the hyperosmotic tubular fluid from the descending limb of the loop of Henle flows into the ascending limb, still more solute is continuously pumped out of the tubules and deposited into the medullary interestitium.
4. These steps are repeated over and over, with the net effect of adding more that more solute to the medulla in excess of water. The process multiplies the 200 mOsm/L concentration gradient established by the active sodium transport out of the thick ascending loop of Henle, eventually raising the interstitial osmolarity to 1200 to 1400 mOsm/L in the pelvic tip of the medulla.

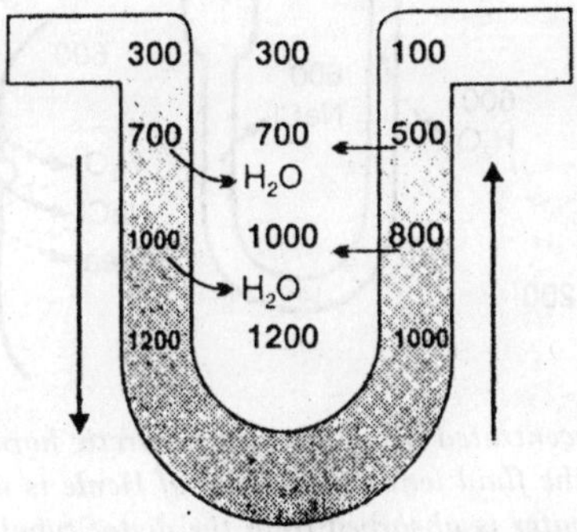

CC Multiplier system in the loop of Henle for producing a hyperosmotic renal medulla (Numerical values are in milliosmoles per litre).

Thus, the repetitive reabsorption of sodium chloride by the thick ascending loop of henle and continued inflow of new NaCl from the PCT into the loop of Henle is called the countercurrent multiplier, The sodium chloride resorbed from the ascending loop of loop of Henle keeps adding to the newly arrived sodium chloride, thus "multiplying" its concentration on the medullary interstitium.

Role of the Distal Tubule and Collecting Ducts in Excreting a Concentrated Urine : When the tubular fluid leaves the loop of Henle and flows into the distal convoluted tubule in the renal cortex the fluid is dilute, with an osmolarity of only about

100 mOsm/L. The early distal tubule further dilutes the tubular fluid because this segment, like the ascending loop of Henle, actively transports sodium chloride out of the tubule but is relatively impermeable to water.

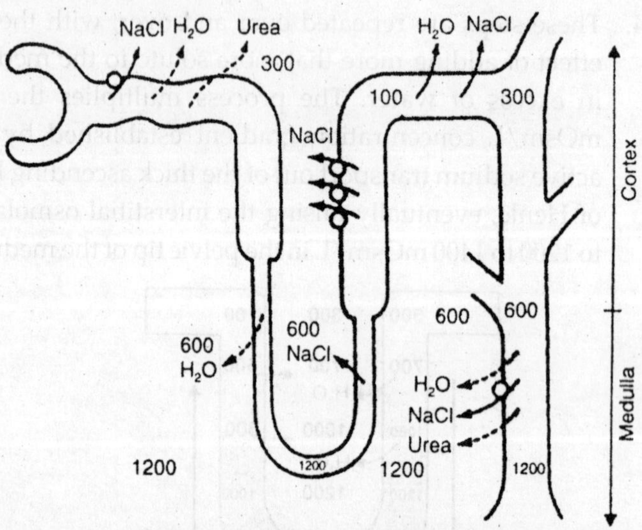

Formation of a concentrated urine when antidiuretic hormone (ADH) levels are high. See that the fluid leaving the loop of Henle is dilute but becomes concentrated as water is absorbed from the distal tubules and collecting tubules. With high ADH levels, the osmolarity of the urine is about the same as the osmolarity of the renal medullary interstitial fluid in the papilla, which is about 1200 mOsm/L. (Numerical values are in milliosmoles per litre).

As fluid flows into the cortical collecting tubule, the amount of water reabsorbed is critically dependent on the plasma concentration of ADH. In the absence of ADH, this segment is almost impermeable to water and fails to reabsorb water but continues to reabsorb solutes and further dilutes the urine. When there is a high concentration of ADH, the cortical collecting tubule becomes highly permeable to water, so that large amounts of water are now reabsorbed from the tubule into the cortex interstitium, where it is swept away by the rapidly flowing peritubular capillaries. *The fact that these large amounts of water are reabsorbed into the cortex, rather than into the renal medulla helps to preserve the high medullary interstitial fluid osmolarity.*

In mammals, the kidney is responsible for monitoring blood pressure and initiating corrective action if the blood pressure begins to drop. In response to several stimuli *e.g.* decreased arterial volume, decreased sodium presentation at the distal tubule, the *juxtaglomerular cells (JG cells)* of the renal cortex (modified smooth muscle cells located in the walls of the afferent and efferent arterioles immediately proximal to the glomeruli) manufacture a proteolytic enzyme renin and secrete it into the blood via the renal vein.

The *macula densa* is a specialized group of epithelial cells in the distal tubules that comes in close contact with the afferent and efferent arterioles. Macula densa cells and *juxtaglomerular cells* in the walls of the afferent and efferent arterioles together constitute the *Juxtaglomerular Complex.* Decreased macula densa sodium chloride causes dilation of afferent arterioles and increased renin release.

In the blood, renin acts upon its specific substrate, an α_2 - globulin that is normally present in blood plasma although it is produced in the liver. This globulin is termed angiotensinogen. From angiotensionogen, the enzyme renin splits off a polypeptide fragment called angiotensin I which is a decapeptide containing 10 amino acids.

Another enzyme called *converting enzyme* in endothelial cells of the capillaries of the lung acts on angiotensin I to split off 2 amino acids (leucine and histidine) and thus to form the octapeptide angiotensin II. The decapeptide angiotensin I is only slightly active. Angiotensin II is the active material, having a pressor activity about 200 times that of norepinephrine. It has three functions :

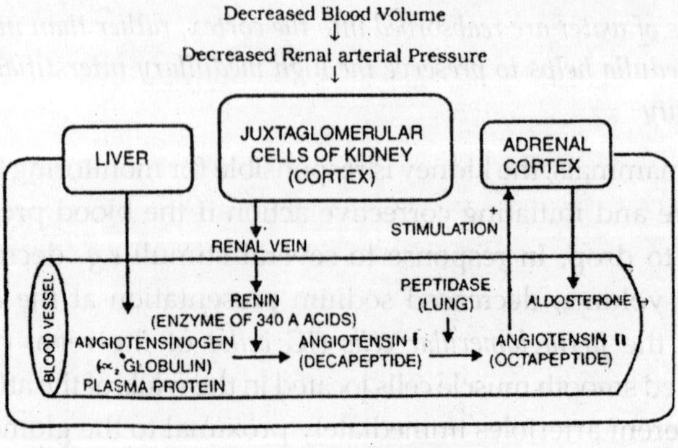

Summary of the Renin–Renin–Angiotensin–Aldosterone System.

As the tubular fluid flows along the medullary collecting ducts, there is further water reabsorption from the tubular fluid into the interstitium, but the total amount of water is relatively small compared with that added to the cortex interstitium. The reabsorbed water is quickly carried away by the vksa recta into the venous blood. When high levels of ADH are present, the collecting ducts become permeable to water, so that the fluid at the end of the collecting ducts has essentially the same osmolarity as the interstitial fluid of the renal medulla—about 1200 mOsm/L. Thus, by reabsorbing as much water as possible, the kidneys form a highly concentrated urine, excreting normal amounts of solutes in the urine while adding water back to the extracellular fluid and compensating for deficits of body water.

Countercurrent Exchange in the Vasa Recta Preserves Hyperosmolarity of the Renal Medullary Interstitium : There are two special features of the renal medullary blood flow that contribute to the preservation of the high solute concentrations:

1. *The medullary blood* flow is low, accounting for only 1 to 2 per cent of the total renal blood flow. This sluggish blood flow is sufficient to supply the metabolic needs of to tissues but helps to minimize solute loss from the medullary interstitium.

2. *The vasa recta serve as countercurrent exchangers,* minimizing washout of solutes from the medullary interstitium.

Blood enters and leaves the medulla by way of the vasa recta at the boundary of the cortex and renal medulla. The *vasa recta,* like other capillaries, are highly permeable to solutes in the blood, except for the plasma proteins. As blood descends into the medulla towards the papillae, it becomes progressively more concentrated, partly by solute entry from the interstitium and partly by loss of water into the interstitium. By the time the blood reaches the tips of the *vasa recta,* it has a concentration of about 1200 mOsm/L, the same as that of the medullary interstitium. As blood ascends back towards the cortex, it becomes progressively less concentrated as solutes diffuse back out into the medullary interstitium and as water moves into the *vasa recta.*

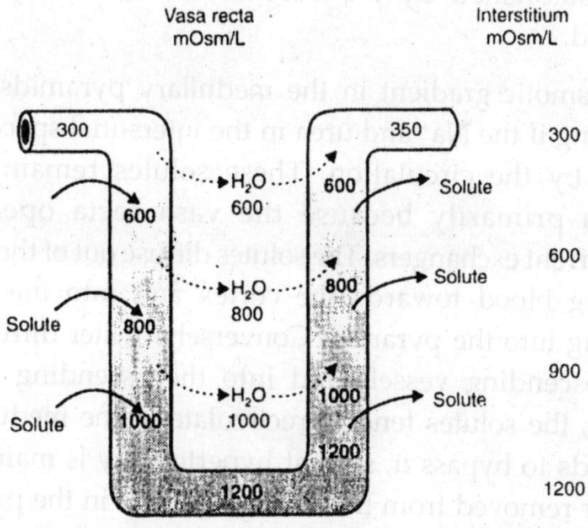

Countercurrent exchange in the vasa recta. Plasma flowing down the descending limb of the vasa recta becomes more hyperosmotic because of diffusion of water out of the blood and diffusion of solutes from the renal interstitial fluid into the blood. In the ascending limb of the vasa recta, salutes diffuse back into the interstitial fluid and water diffuses back into the vasa recta. Large amounts of solutes would be lost from the renal medulla without the U shape of the vasa recta capillaries.

(Numerical values are in millosmoles per litre.)

Thus, although there is a large amount of fluid and solute exchange across the vasa recta, there is little net dilution of the concentration of the interstitial fluid at each level of the renal medulla because of the U shape of the vasa recta calories, which act as countercurrent exchangers. *Thus, the vasa recta do not create the medullary hyperosmolarity, but they do prevent if from being dissipated.*

The U-shaped structure of the vessels minimizes loss of solute from the interstitium but does not prevent the bulk flow of fluid and solutes into the blood through the usually colloid osmotic and hydrostatic pressures that favour reabsorption in these capillaries. Thus, under steadystate conditions, the *vasa recta* carry away only as much solute and water as is absorbed from the medullary tubules, and the high concentration of solutes established by the countercurrent mechanism is maintained.

The osmotic gradient in the medullary pyramids would not last long if the Na^+ and urea in the interstitial spaces were removed by the circulation. These solutes remain in the pyramids primarily because the vasa recta operate as countercurrent exchangers. The solutes diffuse out of the vessels conducting blood towards the cortex and into the vessels descending into the pyramid. Conversely, water diffuses out of the descending vessels and into the ascending vessels. Therefore, the solutes tend to recirculate in the medulla and water tends to bypass it, so that hypertonicity is maintained. The water removed from the collecting ducts in the pyramids is also removed by the vasa recta and enters the general circulation. It should be noted that countercurrent exchange is a passive process; it depends upon diffusion of water and solutes in both directions across the permeable walls of the vasa recta and could not maintain the osmotic gradient along the pyramids if the process of countercurrent multiplication in the loops of Henle were to cease.

Composition of Urine

(1) Water 96%

(2) Urea 2%

(3) Other dissolved solids 2%

(i) *Uric acid* : derived from the nucleic acid metabolism of the body tissues.

(ii) *Creatinine* : an organic by product of muscle

(iii) *Inorganic salts* : chlorides, phosphates, sulfates and oxalates of sodium, potassium and calcium. Small quantities of NH_3, *Urobilin* and *Haematoporphyrin are* also present.

Characteristics of Urine

(1) It is pale yellow (amber) in colour due to the presence of a pigment *urochrome,* which is a breakdown product of haemoglobin.

(2) It is *aromatic* in odour when fresh. The odour becomes *ammoniacal* after bacterial decomposition of urea.

(3) It is slightly *acid* in reaction (pH 6.0).

(4) Its *specific gravity* ranges between 1.001 and 1.04.

(5) A healthy adult passes approximately 1-1½ litres in 24 hours. Urine volume is less in summer or in warm climates for its inversely related to the extend of perspiration.

Nitrogenous end-products, coffee, tea and alcoholic beverages have a diuretic effect.

Abnormal Constituents of Urine

(1) Protein (albumin) in many conditions particularly.

(2) Blood disease or injury of the renal tract.

(3) Sugar (glucose) in Diabetes mellitus.

(4) Ketone bodies (acetoacetic acid, β-Hydroxybutyric acid and acetone) in diabetes and starvation.

(5) Bile in jaundice.

Hormonal Control of Renal Function the Renin-angiotensin-aldosterone System (Renal Pressor System) : In addition to excretory functions, the kidney acts as an endocrine organ, elaborating a variety of hormones which affect other organs and tissues and several substances which may act only locally within the kidney itself.

(1) Angiotensin II increases the force of the heart beat and constricts the arterioles, thus raising blood pressure. In addition, it also brings about contraction of smooth muscle (myotropic effect).

(2) Angiotensin II has a second indirect effect on blood volume and pressure. When it reaches the cells of adrenal cortex, it stimulates them to secret the electrolyte regulating hormone, aldosterone, Aldosterone, by causing retention of sodium (active reabsorption) and water by the kidney tubules, tends to increase the blood volume which in turn, raises the blood pressure and reduces renin production.

(3) Angiotensin II directly stimulates sodium reabsorption in the proximal tubules, the loops of Henle and the distal tubules.

Since angiotensin II Stimulates the adrenal cortex, this effect entitles it to be regarded as an intermediate of tropic *hormone.* Normal kidneys, plasma and to a lesser extent, other tissues contain a proteolytic enzyme called *angiotensinase* which is capable of disturbing angiotensin.

Vasopressin (Pitressin) or Antidiuretic Hormone (ADH) is secreted by the posterior pituitary which controls the permeability to water of the distil convoluted tubules and collecting ducts. The secretion of this hormone is regulated by the water concentration of the blood. Its active secretion leads to the production of a scanty, concentrated urine.

Paratharmone or Parathyroid Hormone (PTH) promotes the absorption of Ca^{2+} in the kidney tubules.

Water Balance

Water Intake : Most of the water taken into the body enters orally, either as plain water or in the form of beverages; and alongwith the food substances. A small amount called *metabolic water* formed in the body, is derived from the oxidation of food stuffs. The quantity of metabolic water (200-300 ml/day) depends on the metabolic rate of the individual.

Water Loss : Water is lost from the body in 4 ways :

(i) as sensible and insensible perspiration from the skin,

(ii) as water vapour in the expired air from lungs.

(iii) as a constituent of faeces from the intestines.

(iv) as urine from the kidney.

The amount of sweat produces a associated with the maintenance of normal body temperature. The amount lost in expired air and in the *faeces is almost constant.* Therefore the balance between intake and output is maintained by the kidneys. Under normal conditions, the minimum urinary output is about 500 ml per day which is essential for the removal of waste materials from the body by this route. The amount of water produced in excess of this is controlled by antidiuretic hormone (ADH) from the posterior pituitary.

Regulation of Water

Pituitary ADH regulates water reabsorption in the distal tubules and collecting ducts aided by the activity of osmoreceptors located in the anterior hypothelamic region of the brain. Osmoreceptors are special cells which are sensitive to changes in the osmotic pressure of the blood.

Increased Osmotic Pressure of Blood : If the osmotic pressure of the blood is raised, the osmo-receptors in the hypohalamus are stimulated and there is an increase in the output of ADH by the pituitary gland. In turn, ADH increases permeability of distal an collecting ducts to water, leading to the production of a scanty, concentrated urine.

INCREASED OSMOTIC PRESSURE OF BLOOD

↓

STIMULATES OSMO-RECEPTORS IN HYPOTHALAMUS

↓

STIMULATE POSTERIOR LOBE OF PITUITARY GLAND

↓

INCREASES ANTIDURETIC HORMONE (ADH) SECRETION

↓

INCREASES PERMEABILITY TO WATER OF DISTAL TUBULES AND COLLECTING DUCTS

↓

INCREASES REABSORPTION OF WATER

↓

(a) SCANTY, CONCENTRATED URINE

↓

(b) REDUCED OSMOIC PRE SSURE OF THE BLOOD

Osmoregulation during high Osmotic Pressure

Reduced Osmotic Pressure of Blood : If the osmotic pressure of the blood is reduced (when it gets diluted) as by the ingestion of large amounts of water, the osmo-receptors are depressed and inhibit pituitary secretion of ADH. The resultant suppression of ADH then permits excretion of more water in the distal and collecting ducts by impairing water-reabsorption. Thus, a large volume of dilute urine results.

REDUCED OSMOTIC PRESSURE OF BLOOD

↓

DECREASES OSMO-RECEPTORS IN HYPOTHALAMUS

↓

INHIBIT POSTERIOR LOBE OF PITUITARY GLAND

↓

DEPRESSES ANTIDURETIC HORMONE (ADH) SECRETION

↓

IMPAIRS PERMEABILITY TO WATER OF DISTAL TUBULES AND COLLECTING DUCTS

↓

INCREASES EXCRETION OF WATER

↓

(a) DILUTE URINE IN LARGE VOLUME

↓

(b) INCREASED OSMOTIC PRESSURE OF THE BLOOD.

Osmoregulation during low osmotic pressure

After deprivation of water, the blood becomes more hypertonic and the osmo-receptors then act to stimulate ADH secretion, which returns more water to the blood in an effort to compensate for the hypertionicity. Under these circumstances, a concentrated urine of small volume results. The cyclic effect maintains the concentration of blood within narrow limits.

A number of drugs, including ingested alcohol, act to suppress ADH secretion and thus to increase, urine flow. On the other hand, certain stresses such as those of surgery or severe trauma, as well as those created by some of the drugs used in anaesthesia, induce excessive production of ADH.

Micturition

Micturition is the act of emptying the bladder or passing urine. From the pelvis of the kidneys, urine is carried down the ureters by peristaltic waves into the urinary bladder. The terminal part of the ureter acts as a sphincter to prevent reflux. The bladder serves to store the urine and to discharge it at convenient intervals. Two refluxes are involved in bladder-control : (1) the storage reflex, which permits the bladder to fill and (2) the voiding reflex, which empties it.

After infancy, the micturition which is primarily a reflex act can be consciously controlled by impulses from the higher centres of the brain.

Physiology of Excretion

The elimination of waste products from the body is called excretion. Strictly speaking, it refers to the removal of the waste products of metabolism, which comprise carbon dioxide, water and nitrogenous wastes. But the removal of CO_2 is a function of the respiratory process. Because there is more than one route for the passage of water, excretion is thought of as the removal of nitrogenous wastes like ammonia, urea or uric acid, etc. Other waste products of protein metabolism may be *Trimethylamine Oxide* (TMO, formed in marine teleosts) and *Guanine* (found in spiders). Allantoin, Allantonic acid, Hippuric acid, Ornithuric acid, Creatine, Creatinine, Purines, Pyrimidines and Pterines are other miscellaneous nitrogenous compounds that are also excreted in small amounts by various animals.

Excretion in Invertebrates

In most unicellular organisms, excretion is simply a process of diffusion through the cell membrane into the surrounding medium (water). In others contractile vacuole may also help in excretion. Essentially the same plan of excretion is employed by sponges and coelenterates, in which the waste is either diffused through the epidermal cells to the surrounding water or into the canals and gastrovascular cavity by the endodermal cells. In the flatworms, there are definite excretory organs, the *flame cells* (protonephridia) which are connected to a branched system of tubes that discharge the waste to the outside.

In annelids, there are nephridia to remove the waste matter collected in the coelomic fluid. Insects have many *malpighian tubules* which pick up waste substances from the body by diffusion and pass them into the digestive tracts. In other arthropods, especially the crustaceans, the excretion is performed by a pair of antennary or maxillary glands. Molluscs have one of more pairs of kidneys or nephridia that remove the wastes from the coelom and the blood. In echinoderms, excretion is affected by amoebocytes.

Excretion in Vertebrates

The following organs are concerned with ridding the body of wastes :

(a) *Skin* : that removes excess water, salts and CO_2

(b) *Lungs* : that remove CO_2 and water.

(c) *Liver* : that excretes bile pigments.

(d) *Alimentary canal* : that removes certain salts.

(e) *Gills :* that remove excess salts in marine fishes.

(f) *Salt glands :* of some marine-birds and the reptiles.

(g) *Kidneys* : that remove excess water, nitrogenous wastes, salts and other materials in the form of urine. The kidneys and associated organs which function in the production and elimination of urine are collectively called the *urinary system.* The latter, in humans and other mammals, takes the major burden (about 75-80%) of excreting the wastes.

Excretory System of Vertebrates

The urinary system is almost similar in all vertebrates. It consists of two kidneys located postero-dorsally. From each kidney a *ureter*, or excretory duct, carries the urine posteriorly. In elasmobranches, amphibians, reptiles and birds these ureters open directly into the cloaca, which is provided with a urinary bladder in some of them. In most mammals, the ureters empty into the bladder which opens to the outside through the *urethra*

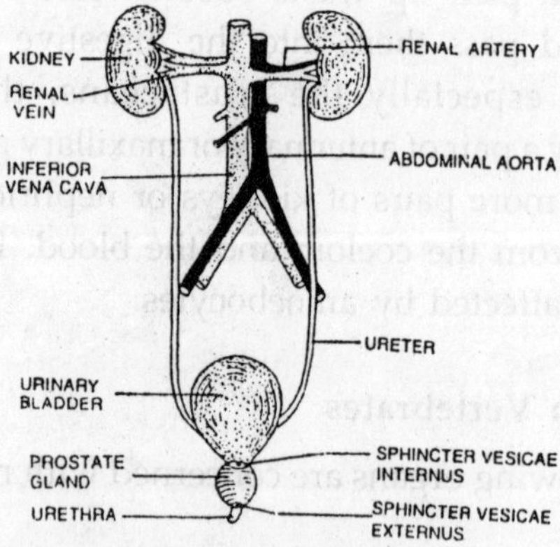

The excretory system of man.

Functional Anatomy of Kidney

In humans the paired kidneys are bean-shaped, each weighing about 4 ounces, and are located just below the stomach, one on each side of the mid-dorsal line. Histologically, each kidney is made up of an outer zone, the *cortex*, and an inner zone, the *medulla*, including its connective tissue and rich vascular supply. Each kidney contains about one million single units called *nephrons*.

Each nephron which is about 45 to 65 mm long consists of a round malpighian body, which is filled- with capillary network called the *glomerulus,* and a tube which is divided into three parts—*the proximal convoluted tubule* (15 mm long and 55 μm in diameter), a *thin segment* (2 to 14 mm long), and the *distal convoluted tubule* (about 5 mm long), which joins with other tubules to form the collecting ducts that open into the *pelvis* of the kidney. Part of the tubule, including the thin segment, makes a hairpin loop which is called the *loop of Henle.* This greatly elongated and narrow loop is adapted specifically for water recovery by means of a countercurrent osmotic multiplier system. Only animals that have the loop of Henle can excrete urine hypertonic to their blood.

The entire kidney tubule is surrounded by blood capillaries. From the pelvis, the ureter leads to the bladder where the urine is temporarily stored. The blood flow to the kidney is very great. In a resting adult, the kidneys receive about 1.2-1.3 litre of blood per minute.

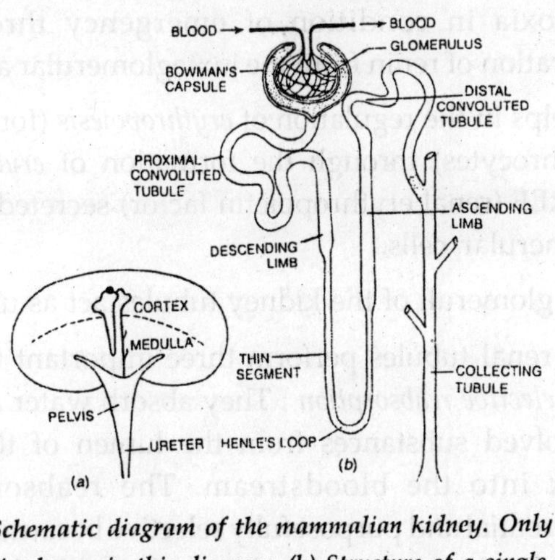

(a) *Schematic diagram of the mammalian kidney. Only one nephron is shown in this diagram,* (b) *Structure of a single nephron.*

Functions of the Kidney

1. It excretes waste products, especially the nitrogenous and sulphur containing end products of protein metabolism.

2. It helps to maintain the normal hydrogen-ion concentration of body fluids and electrolytes.
3. It helps to maintain water balance of the body and thereby plasma volume.
4. It helps to maintain the optimum concentration of certain constituents of blood (by the process of selective reabsorption).
5. It eliminates drugs and various toxic substances from the body.
6. It manufactures certain new substances like ammonia, hippuric acid and inorganic phosphates. Ammonia helps in keeping the acid-base equilibrium.
7. It helps in maintaining the osmotic pressures in blood and tissues.
8. It helps in the regulation of blood pressure during hypoxia in condition of emergency through the liberation of renin from the juxtaglomerular apparatus.
9. It helps in the regulation of *erythropoiesis* (formation of erythrocytes) through the formation of *erythropoietin* by REF (renal erythropoietin factor) secreted from the glomerular cells.
10. The glomeruli of the kidney tubules act as ultrafilters.
11. The renal tubules perform three important functions: *(a) Selective reabsorption* : They absorb water and other dissolved substances from the lumen of the tubule back into the bloodstream. The reabsorption is differential and purposefully selective because the more useful substances are reabsorbed to a higher degree than the less useful ones, *(b) Tubular secretion :* Tubules not only reabsorb but can also actively transfer certain substances from the bloodstream into the lumen of tubules, (c) *Formation of some new substances*: The tubular

epithelium can also form certain new substances such as ammonia, inorganic phosphates, etc.

Endocrine Function of the Kidney

The endocrine function of the kidney is very important. Besides *erythropoietin*, which stimulates production of erythrocytes in the bone marrow, kidneys secrete several other important hormonal products. *Prostaglandins*, which are produced in the kidney as well as in several other tissues, have a variety of effects on renal function.

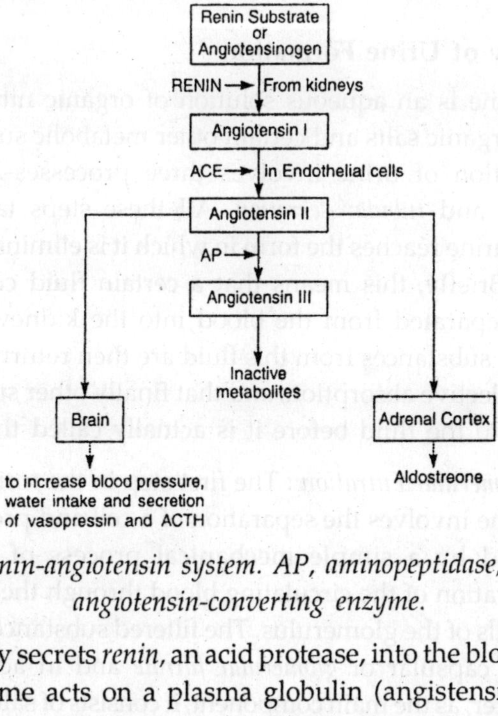

The renin-angiotensin system. AP, aminopeptidase; ACE, angiotensin-converting enzyme.

Kidney secrets *renin*, an acid protease, into the bloodstream. This enzyme acts on a plasma globulin (angistensinogen) to form angiotensin I which, by the action of angiotensin-converting enzyme (ACE), is converted to angiotensin II. Angiotensin II acts directly on the adrenal cortex to increase the secretion of *aldosterone*. Thus, renin-angiotensin system is a major regulator of aldosterone secretion. Angiotensin II also acts on the brain to increase blood pressure, water intake and secretion of vasopressin and ACTH.

The final step in the synthesis of the steroid 1,15-*Dihydroxycholecalciferol* or calcitriol 1,25-$(OH)_2D_3$ occurs in the kidney. It is the active metabolite of vitamin D that has important regulatory actions on phosphate and calcium metabolism. Several *kinins,* bradykinin, lysylbradykinin or kalidin, which are potent vasodilator peptides, are also produced in the kidney. They have several important effects on renal function such as renal circulation as well as on renal sodium and water excretion.

Physiology of Urine Formation

The urine is an aqueous solution of organic nitrogenous wastes, inorganic salts and certain other metabolic substances. The formation of urine involves three processes-*.filtration, reabsorption* and *tubular secretion.* All these steps take place before the urine reaches the form in which it is eliminated from the body. Briefly, this means that a certain fluid containing wastes is separated from the blood into the kidney tubules, that certain substances from this fluid are then returned to the blood by selective absorption, and that finally other substances are added to the fluid before it is actually called the urine.

(a) *Glomerular Filtration* : The first step in the formation of urine involves the separation of a cell and protein-free fluid by a simple mechanical process of pressure filtration of the circulating blood through the capillary walls of the glomerulus. The filtered substance is called the capsular or *glomerular filtrate* and in addition to water, as the main component, it consists of salts, sugars, urea, uric acid and some other substances. This process of filtration is produced by the force of excess blood pressure in the glomerular capillaries over the osmotic pressure of the blood colloids. The hydrostatic pressure in the glomerular capillary is estimated to be about 70 mm Hg, which is considerably higher than in capillaries elsewhere. The blood osmotic pressure is about 28 mm Hg. There is a back pressure, *i.e.*, a hydrostatic pressure, in the capsule and tubule of about 10 mm Hg. Thus, the *effective glomerular filtration pressure is* equal to about 32 mm Hg. [70- (28 + 10)].

There are so many glomeruli involved in this process so that the average glomerular filtrate formed by a normal adult is about 125 ml per minute, or 170-180 litres per day. It has been found by *Prof. Richards* (1938) that the filtrate contains the same composition of dissolved substances as plasma except for the absence of proteins.

Quantification of the *glomerular filtration rate* (GFR) helps in understanding how various substances are handled by the kidney. The GFR in normal man is about 125 ml/min. Thus, substances whose excretory rates are less than their filtration rates must undergo net tubular reabsorption, whereas substances whose excretory rates are more than their filtration rates must undergo net secretion.

The term *clearance* is generally used to quantify the removal of a substance from the blood during its passage through the kidneys. It is defined as the equivalent volume of blood plasma that contains all of a particular substance excreted in the urine in 1 minute. It is expressed as $C = UV/P$ where C is clearance in ml per minute, *U* is concentration in urine, V is urine volume in ml per minute, and *P* is plasma concentration. The clearance of a substance that has a concentration in plasma identical with that in the glomerular filtrate and is neither reabsorbed nor secreted by the tubular epithelium is a measure of the rate of glomerular filtration.

The substance that most nearly meets these requirements is *inulin*, a polymer of fructose found in the roots of certain plants. Other materials that have been used are creatinine and radioisotopes of vitamin B_{12}. All of these yield clearance values of about 100 to 125 ml per minute per 1.73 m^2 of surface area in human males and somewhat lower values in females.

As noted above any substance that is completely filtered, has a clearance less than that of inulin, and is not bound to plasma protein must be *reabsorbed* as the glomerular filtrate flows through the tubules. Such substances are primarily Na^+, K^+, Cl^-, water, glucose, urea, amino acids, and uric acid. And any substance whose clearance is more than that of inulin must be *secreted* into the urine by tubular cells. $NH4^+$, H^+, and N^{1}-methyl-nicotinamide behave in this manner as do some other subtances like penicillin, p-amino hippurate (PAH), and phenolsulfon-phthalein. The ratio of inulin to PAH clearance is termed the *filtration fraction* and is approximately 18 per cent in normal individuals.

Another parameter of renal excretory function is the *transport maximum* (Tm), which is the maximum ability of the kidneys either to reabsorb or to secrete a given material. For example, since no glucose is excreted when the plasma glucose concentration is 100 mg/dl, the kidneys must absorb 125 mg of glucose per minute in the proximal tubules. However, at an artificially elevated plasma glucose concentration of 400 mg/dl, that is, a glomerular filtration rate for glucose of 500 mg/minute, 200 mg/ minute of glucose may be excreted. The difference (300 mg/minute) is the maximum rate at which the kidneys can reabsorb glucose and is denoted as *Tm* for glucose.

(b) *Selective Reabsorption* : As the glomerular filtrate passes along the renal tubule from Bowman's capsule, most of its water and some of the dissolved substances are continuously reabsorbed through the walls of the tubule into the blood of the surrounding capillaries. Thus, in passing along the proximal convoluted tubule alone, about 85% of water, Na^+, Cl^-, HCO_3- and glucose of the glomerular filtrate are reabsorbed into the blood. As a result of further selective reabsorption in loop of

Henle and the distal convoluted tubule only about 1% of the original filtrate is left.

The substances that are absorbed in large amount (water and glucose) are called *high-threshold substances.* Others, like urea, uric acid and certain salts, that are partly absorbed and partly excreted are called *low-threshold substances,* and still others that are not absorbed at all are known as *non-threshold substances.* It is believed that an active transport mechanism operates in the reabsorption process.

The location of reabsorption of each substance varies. Some are primarily reabsorbed in the proximal tubule, some in the distal, and others are reabsorbed in part by both. The glucose, phosphate, bicarbonate, potassium, sodium, amino acids, and protein are reabsorbed in the proximal tubule. In the distal tubule, chloride and more sodium are reabsorbed.

Sodium is absorbed in the proximal tubule by a variety of *co-transport systems.* An important chracteristic of such systems is the interdependence of the transport of Na^+ and the co-transported solute. Thus, neither Na^+ nor the solute is efficiently transported without the other, and each enhances transport of the other. The high intracellular concentrations of various solutes such as glucose and amino acids established by these active transport processes drive the passive extrusion of these materials from the particular border of the cells.

The carriers mediating such transport are envisaged as having distinct binding sites for Na^+ and the co-transported solute. Several such carriers exist in the lumenal border of the renal epithelial cells, each of which simultaneously transports Na^+ together with a specific solute such as glucose, amino acids, phosphate, or lactate. Separate systems exist for each solute or class of solute. These are examples of *secondary active transport systems.* The energy for these transport systems is ultimately derived from a Na^+, K^+ - ATPase located in the epithelial cell's basolateral plasma membrane. This system accomplishes primary active transport of Na^+, extruding Na^+ from the cell while bringing K^+ in, thus maintaining the Na^+ gradient responsible for the functioning of the co-transport systems. It extrudes three Na^+ in exchange for two K^+ that are pumped into the cell.

Reabsorption of glucose by the Na co-transport system is normally complete in the proximal tubule. The presumed carrier shows stereo specificity for D-glucose. It is the carrier-mediated nature of glucose transport that accounts for the phenomenon of *transport maximum*, discussed above. When the *Tm* for glucose is exceeded as a result of hyperglycemia, as in diabetes mellitus, glucose appears in the urine.

(c) *Tubular Secretion* : The renal tubules are capable of transporting substances from the blood into the filtrate, as well as from the filtrate back into the blood. This process is termed tubular secretion. The active transport process in this instance is more or less similar to that occuring in the reabsorption as previously indicated, except for the differences in direction and specificity of the materials being transferred. Tubular secretion, by contributing to the excretory function of the nephron, increases the overall efficiency in extracting the waste products from the blood.

The final changes in the composition and volume of urine occur in the loop of Henle and the distal convoluted tubule. They are attained through further reabsorption of water and various dissolved substances and through tubular secretion into the filtrate of certain materials including *potassium*, *ammonia* and *hydrogen ions*. In effect, the cells composing the walls of the tubule are responsible for a two-way traffic between the filtrate and blood of the surrounding capillaries. On the one hand, most of the water as well as the essential food materials are reabsorbed from the tubular fluid and restored to the bloodstream. On the other hand, the wastes are removed from the blood by tubular secretion and added to the concentrated filtrate which soon becomes the urine.

Another example of a Na^+ co-transport system that participates in Na^+ reabsorption in the proximal tubule is the process that accomplishes the linked exchange of Na^+ for H^+. This process functions as an *antiport,* Na^+ and H^+ moving in opposite directions. The energy for H^+ secretion into the lumen is derived from the coupled influx of Na^+ down its electrochemical gradient into the cell. Such proton secretion into the tubular lumen leads to net HCO_3- reabsorption. In addition to the Na^+ -H^+ antiport system, which accomplishes an electrically neutral Na^+ - H^+ exchange in the proximal tubules, *active secretion of* H^+ may also be achieved by mechanisms that are not directly coupled to Na^+ transport and are *electrogenic.* This means that a potential difference is established by the H^+ secretion and the rate of the secretory process is in turn influenced by electrical forces. This mechanism appears to predominate in the *collecting duct,* which is capable of generating a large proton gradient and lowering urinary pH. The active H^+ secretion is mediated by ion sensitive ATPases that are distinct from Na^+, K^+ - ATPase.

Both H^+ and K^+ secretion by the distal tubule are accomplished by exchange for Na^+. Although not directly coupled or competitive with one another the transport processes in the distal tubule for H^+ and K^+ do seem to be related in some way. K^+ and H^+ are the two major cations available for secretion in exchange for Na^+, which is reabsorbed. Factors that decrease the abundance of cellular protons lead to decreased urine acidification and increased K^+ secretion. In proximal tubular cells, an active carrier-mediated process is responsible for the secretion of a variety of organic anions. Some endogenous substances secreted by this system include hippurate, bile salts, oxalate, urate and cyclic AMP. Exogenous substances that are secreted by this process include para-aminohippurate (PAH) and a variety of drugs such as penicillin, probenecid, salicylate, saccharin, and several diuretics. Since all of the organic anions share the same carrier (s), their transport is competitive. For example, probenecid inhibits the secretion of penicillin.

It is worth noting that in the overall formation of urine the glomeruli play a passive role since the energy of filtration is supplied by the heart via the pressure of blood. In the subsequent reabsorption and tubular secretion processes, energy is provided by the metabolism of tubule cells.

Countercurrent Theory of Urine Concentration : The quality of mammalian kidney to form a concentrated urine can be attributed to the kidney's *loop of Henle.* This new concept is called the *countercurrent theory* or mechanism, because the scheme of the nephron arrangement of the loop of Henle and the collecting tubule forms a hairpin bend in which the direction of current flow is in opposite or counter directions. Between these opposing currents there appears to be an exchange of water and some solutes. In any one place along the loop the concentration difference between the ascending limb and the descending limb is moderate, but along the length of the loop this moderate concentration difference is additive *i.e.*, there is a multiplication effect. The entire system is, therefore, called a *countercurrent multiplier system.*

New sampling methods have made possible the exact determinations of the fluid content from the different parts of the kidney tubule. These determinations have shown that in comparison with the blood plasma glomerular filtrate is isotonic, the tubular fluid is hypertonic at the tip of Henle's loop, isotonic or even hypotonic at the distal convoluted tubule and hypertonic in the collecting duct. To account for these differences in urine toniciry a countercurrent multiplier mechanism has been proposed. According to this scheme, there is an active transfer of sodium ions from the ascending limb of Henle (which is impermeable to water) to the interstitial tissue. Some of the sodium will now diffuse from its higher tissue concentration to the descending limb, so that there is a gradual increase in salt concentration, until the fluid enters the ascending limb where the same amount of salt is transported back to the tissue again. By this mechanism, sodium is constantly removed from the ascending limb and returned to the descending limb of the loop. As the fluid leaves the loop of Henle or the distal convoluted tubule and enters the collecting duct, the high concentration of salt in the interstitial tissue will draw water from the filtrate in the collecting ducts, and thus the urine is concentrated to its final form.

The new concept indicates also that the degree of urine concentration depends upon the length of the loop of Henle and the collecting tubule. The longer the loop, the higher the urine concentration that can be achieved. The poikilothermic vertebrates lack the loop structure in their kidney tubules and are, therefore, unable to form a urine more concentrated than their blood, because the loop structure is essential to this process.

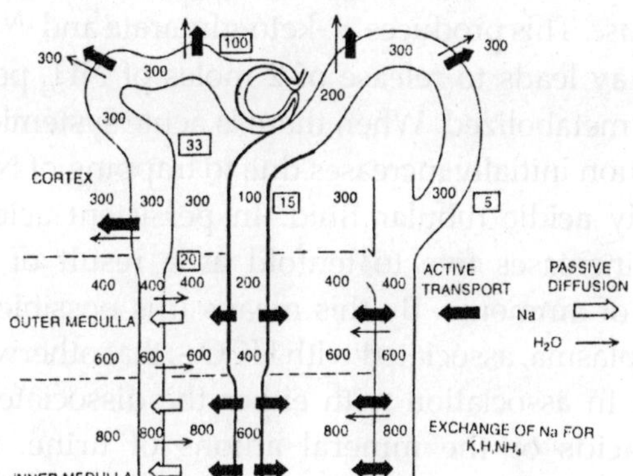

Mechnism of urine formation. The movement of water and sodium is indicated. The numbers in boxes indicate the estimated percentage of glomerular filtrate remaining within the tubule at each level. Concentration of tubularurine or particular fluid are expressed in mOsm/litre.

Acid-base Balance

The excretion of *hydrogen ions* and *ammonia* in varying amounts by the cells of both the proximal and distal convoluted tubules increases or decreases the acidity of urine. Thus, it is an important mechanism in the control of the acidity and basicity of the body tissues and fluids. The kidney, in fact, rids the body of excess acid in several ways. Not only does it excrete a small amount of free hydrogen ions, but most of the excess acid is first neutralized in the kidney tissue itself before being excreted. This is accomplished through the formation of ammonia and phosphate salts. Ammonia is produced in renal epithelial cells largely by the deamination of glutamine taken up from the arterial blood.

$$\text{Glutamine} + H_2O \xrightarrow{\text{glutaminase}} \text{Glutamate} + NH_4^+$$

$$\text{Glutamate} \xrightarrow{\text{glutamic dehydrogenase}} \alpha\text{-ketoglutarate} + NH_4^+$$

The reaction is catalyzed by a mitochondrial enzyme, the phosphate dependent *glutaminase.* The glutamate formed is metabolized within the mitochondria largely by *glutamate dehydrogenase.* This produces α-keto-glutarate and NH_{4+}. Thus, this pathway leads to release of 2 moles of NH_3 per mole of glutamine metabolized. When there is acute systemic acidosis, NH_3 excretion initially increases due to trapping of NH_4^+ in the increasingly acidic tubular fluid. In persistent acidosis NH_3 excretion increases five to tenfold as a result of increased formation of ammonia. By this means it is possible to return Na^+ to the plasma, associated with HCO_3^-, that otherwise would be present in association with either the dissociated fraction of weak acids or the mineral anions of urine. Only this mechanism can compensate for acidosis due to the accumulation of anions of strong acids. Thus, conservation of Na^+ by the renal mechanisms serves to maintain both the alkaline reserve and the volume of plasma. Sometime failure of the NH_4^+-forming mechanism, as in pyelonephritis, may itself be the cause of acidosis.

Control of Renal Function

The formation of urine is the result of two processes *i.e.*, glomerular filtration and tubular modification. The glomerular filtration depends upon the resultant between hydrostatic and osmotic pressures. A fall in the *arterial blood pressure* decreases urine flow primarily by decreasing the glomerular filtration rate due to lowered filtration pressure. When the mean arterial blood pressure decreases below about 60 mm Hg, the urine formation is ceased. A change in resistance in the afferent and efferent arterioles can maintain normal renal function in the face of elevated arterial blood pressure. The afferent and efferent arterioles are capable of independent alterations to control glomerular filtration pressure and renal flow. By virtue of these adjustments, the kidney can usually maintain normal function despite considerable circulatory changes in the rest of the body.

In order to maintain the constancy of body fluid volume, the kidneys are able to vary the volume of urine output. As mentioned above, over a wide range of arterial blood pressures, the pressure within the glomeruli is maintained constant, but if the arterial pressure falls much below 60 or 70 mm Hg, the glomerular filtration is ceased as does the formation of urine. This is an extreme event. Under more normal circumstances glomerular filtration remains constant and urine output is regulated by the amount of water reabsorbed. Mechanisms of *glomerulotubular balance and tubuloglomerular feed back* are shown in Fig.

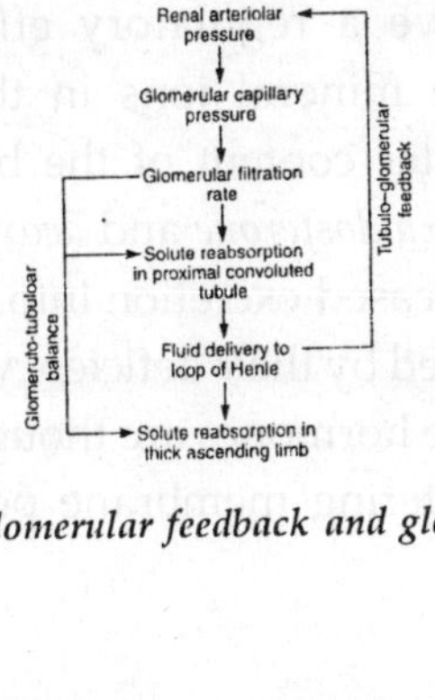

Mechanisms of tubuloglomerular feedback and glomerulotubular balance.

The main regulation of urine output is achieved by the antidiuretic hormone and also by the adrenocortical hormones.

Hormonal Control of Excretion

In mammals, the urine production is controlled by water-retaining principles and some aderno-cortical hormones. The *antidiuretie hormone* (ADH) or *vasopressin* is produced by the supraoptic nucleus of the hypothalamus and passes along the infundibular stalk to the neurohypophysis or the posterior pituitary gland where it is stored. It reaches the kidney through the bloodstream and promotes the reabsorption of water by the distal convoluted tubules and the collecting tubules.

It is quite interesting that the secretion of the ADH varies with the intake of water. If less water is taken more ADH is produced to decrease the volume of urine, or if more water is taken less ADH is secreted so that only a small amount of water is reabsorbed and the excess is allowed to go in urine. The neurohypophyseal hormone of the amphibians also works like the mammalian ADH.

It has been suggested that the neurohypophyseal hormone reduces the volume of urine by two means : firstly by reduction in filtration due to constriction of glomerular arterioles, and secondly by increasing the tubular reabsorption of water.

Other hormones affecting excretion are the aderno-cortical hormones. They have a regulatory effect on the relative concentration of the mineral ions in the body fluids and therefore, on the water content of the body. The important mineral corticoids are *aldosterone* and *deoxycorticosterone.* Their lack results in an increased excretion into the urine of Na^+, Cl^- and water accompanied by their deficiency in the blood. Recent work shows that these hormones are thought to have a diuretic effect probably by altering membrane permeability.

Excretion of Nitrogenous Waste Products

In living organisms the major nitrogen-containing substances are never completely metabolized to yield free nitrogen. But nitrogen-containing end products like *ammonia*, *urea* and *uric acid* are formed. Depending on the chief nitrogenous excretory product, the animals may be divided into three main groups as follows :

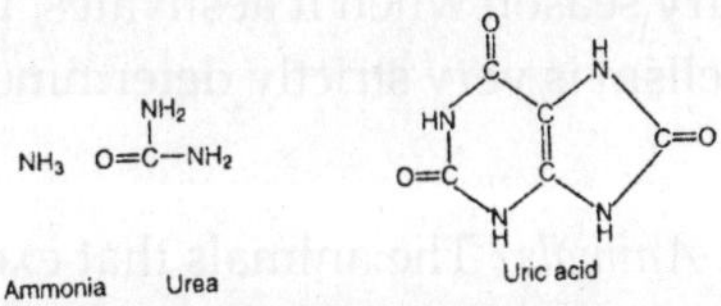

Nitrogen-containing end products of protein metabolism.

(a) *Ammonotelic Animals* : The animals that excrete nitrogen in the form of ammonia are called ammonotelic. The chief chemocal state in which metabolic nitrogenous waste products are axcreted by different animals depends upon the given species and the evolutionary adaptations animals living in water are ammonotelic, for they can excrete ammonia as such into the surrounding water without converting it to the less toxic form of urea or uric acid. Thus, most aquatic invertebrates and freshwater fishes are, in general, ammonotelic as they have an unlimited supply of water at their disposal into which ammonia is rapidly diffused from their bodies. In protozoa, the quantity of ammonia excreted varies with diet, stage in culture cycle and species. Echinoderms are ammonotelic, but they also give off considerable amounts of amino acids. Polychaete worms are ammonotelic. However, urea and traces of uric acid are reported in *Arenicola's* coelomic fluid. The cephalopods, *Sepia* and *Octopus*, excrete most of their nitrogen as NH_3 and the pelecypods and some gastropods are also ammonotelic.

Freshwater fish are ammonotelic, although they also excrete some urea. Many of the marine teleosts are ammonotelic, but also excrete considerable amounts of urea and other products like trimethylamine oxide (TMO). The latter is a soluble nontoxic substance. However, the fact that *ammonotelism* is definitely related to the habitat and the mode of life, can be illustrated by citing the example of the African lung fish, *Protopterus.* It produces ammonia when there is abundant supply of water. But during the dry season when it aestivates, it produces urea. Thus, ammonotelism is very strictly determined by the supply of water.

(b) *Ureotelic Animals* : The animals that excrete nitrogen in the form of urea are called ureotelic. Terrestrial animals have limited supply of water and cannot get rid of ammonia unless it is converted into more complex and less toxic compounds. In ureotelic animals (e.g., elasmobranchs, amphibians and mammals), urea is formed in the liver from the nitrogen of amino acids and then excreted by the kidney. But in these animals also some water is required to dissolve urea so that it may be excreted with the urine. Thus, a change from ammonotelic to ureotelic appears to be closely correlated with the supply of water. When water is plentiful, the tadpole of frog is ammonotelic. But as it metamorphoses and leaves water, it becomes ureotelic.

Mammals including monotremes, are ureotelic. Their embryonic life is more or less aquatic and the embryonic wastes diffuse rapidly into the maternal circulation. However, there is need for conservation of water in adult mammals, and urea may be concentrated by as much as a hundred times by the reabsorption of water in the kidney tubules. According to *Schmidt-Nielsen* (1952), in desert animals like the kangaroo rat *(Dipodomys),* and possibly in other mammals depending on high protein and low water intake, there may be active tubular secretion of urea. Ruminants can use urea as an ultimate protein source, and on a low protein diet a camel or sheep can reduce its urea excretion twenty fold and can retain injected urea for use in the lumen.

(c) *Uricotelic Animals* : The animals are referred to as uricotelic when they excrete nitrogen in the form of uric acid. The excretion of uric acid by uricotelic forms is the last step in the course of the biochemical evolution of nitrogen excretion. Since uric acid is almost insolube, its excretion is definitely advantageous over the previous methods. Terrestrial reptiles and birds are, therefore, uricotelic. In these organisms uric acid is excreted by the kidney tubules directly into the tubular urine. It precipiates out of solution, leaving the water free to be reabsorbed and is finally released as a white paste. The urine formed in the malpighian tubules of insects is rich in uric acid and there may be a mass of uric acid crystals left after absorption of water from the secreted solution.

The formation of uric acid may be even more important in the development of the embryo than in conserving the water of the adult. All animals that produce uric acid from amino acids deposit eggs outside the maternal organism. Since the embryo must develop on the limited supply of water present in the egg, it would be better if the excretory products are deposited as insoluble substance. Thus, it can be concluded that the chief nitrogenous excretory product of an organism appears to be closely correlated with the supply of water, especially during the embryonic development.

Thus, it is quite clear from the description of ammonotelic, ureotelic and uricotelic animals, that the nitrogen excretion is a labile character. It has changed during the evolution of several groups according to their habitat and a *relationship exists between nitrogen excretion and evolutionary adaptations of animals.* In some animals the excretory pattern is changed with the life cycle. In others, changes in nitrogen excretion may be induced by the diet, availability of water, and osmotic stress, etc.

Besides proteins many other compounds contain nitrogen. Among these are the nucleic acids, which in humans give rise to the uric acid that is present in a small amount in the urine. In other mammals, the uric acid is transformed by an enzyme to allantoin. The latter is further broken down to urea in many amphibians and fishes. However, in aquatic invertebrates ammonia is frequently the end product of the nucleic acid metabolism.

Method of Urea Formation

The best known method of formation of urea from the ammonia of protein metabolism is by the *Omithine cycle.* The urea is formed principally in the liver, then it enters the bloodstream and is eventually excreted by the kidney.

The first step involves the enzymatic reaction whereby CO_2, NH_3 and ATP, in the presence of a certain derivative of glutamic acid, are converted to the compound *carbamyl phosphate,* ADP and H_3PO_4. The compound in turn reacts with the amino acid *omithine* in the presence of a suitable enzyme to form the amino acid *Citrulline*. The next two enzymatic steps lead to the formation of the amino acid *arginine* whereby citrulline and aspartic acid react in the presence of ATP are form first *arginino-succinic acid* which is then converted to arginine and fumaric acid.

Thus, aspartic acid provides one of its amino groups to citrulline to form arginine. Some of the arginine may subsequently be used for protein synthesis, whereas some may be broken down by the hydrolyzing enzyme *arginase* to yield urea and one of the starting materials, omithine, thus completing the urea cycle. In this way two moles of NH_3 (one via aspartic acid and the other via carbamyl phosphate), one CO_2 and 3 moles of ATP are used in the cycle to form one molecule of urea. The complete cycle is shown in Fig. and the sequece of reactions is given as follows :

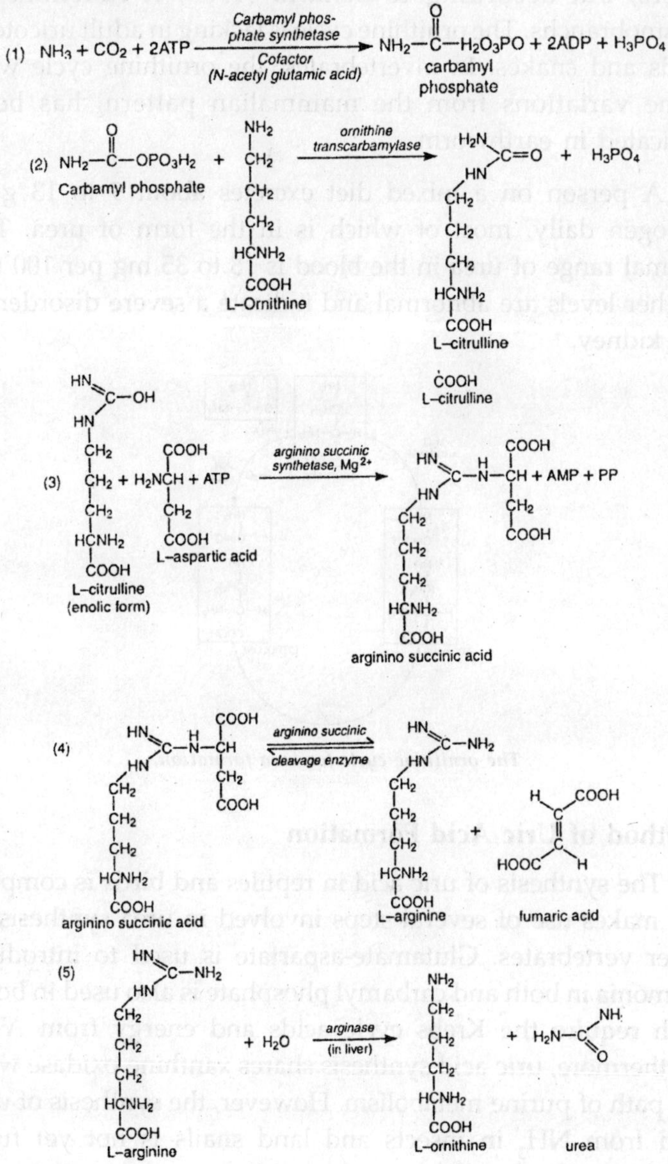

The ornithine cycle operates in the livers of mammals, frogs and turtles. The cycle is said to be absent in the teleost livers, but according to *Baldwin* (1960) it functions in elasmobranchs. The ornithine cycle is lacking in adult uricotelic birds and snakes. In invertebrates, the ornithine cycle with some variations from the mammalian pattern, has been indicated in earthworm.

A person on a mixed diet excretes about 9 to 13 g of nitrogen daily, most of which is in the form of urea. The normal range of urea in the blood is 18 to 35 mg per 100 ml. Higher levels are abnormal and indicate a severe disorder of the kidney.

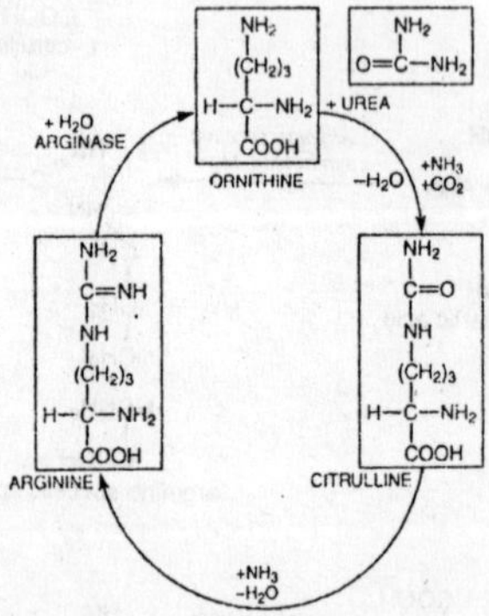

The ornithine cycle for urea formation.

Method of Uric Acid Formation

The synthesis of uric acid in reptiles and birds is complex but makes use of several steps involved in urea synthesis in other vertebrates. Glutamate-aspartate is used to introduce ammonia in both and carbamyl phosphate is also used in both. Both require the Krebs cycle acids and energy from ATP. Furthermore, uric acid synthesis shares xanthine oxidase with the path of purine metabolism. However, the synthesis of uric acid from NH_3 in insects and land snails is not yet fully explained.

Bibliography

Asdell, S.A. : *Patterns of Mammalian Reproduction,* Comstock, New York, 1946.

Assali, N.S. : *Biology of Gestation,* Academic Press, New York, 1968.

Bahr, G.F. : *Chromosomes and Chromatin Structure,* Academic Press, New York, 2001.

Bell, G.H. and Davidson J.N. : *Textbook of Physiology,* John Wiley, London, 1985.

Bendall, J.R. : *Muscles, Molecules and Movement,* Heinemann Educational Books, London 1969.

Benjamin, Gutfreud : *Enzymes : Physical Principals,* John Wiley, London, 1972.

Benjamin, Schroeder : *The Primary Structure of Proteins,* John Wiley, London, 1968.

Bernhard, : *The Structure and Function of Enzymes,* Routledge, New York, 1968.

Biggs, R. and Macfarlane, R.G. : *Human Blood Coagulation and its Disorders,* New York, 1962.

Bloomfield, Crothers and Tinoco : *Physical Chemistry of Nucleic Acids,* Harper and Row, London, 1974.

Bogert, L.J. and Calloway D.H. : *Nutrition and Physical Fitness,* Saunders, London, 1973.

Bourne, G.H. : *The Structure and Function of Nervous Tissue,* Academic Press, New York, 1968.

Boyd, J.D. and Hamilton, W.J. : *The Human Placenta,* Cambridge, London, 1978.

Boyer : *The Enzymes,* Academic Press, New York, 1970.

Brambell, F.W.R : *Ovarian Changes in Marshall's Physiology,* John Wiley, London, 1991.

Brohek, J.R. : *Best and Taylor's Physiological Basis of Medical Practice,* Williams & Wilkins, New York, 1973.

Burton, B.T. : *Heinz Handbook of Nutriton,* McGraw Hill, New York, 1965.

Castillo, J. : *Progress in Biophysics and Biophysical Chemistry,* Prentice Hall, London, 1956.

Crampton, E.W. : *Fundamentals of Nutrition,* W.H. Freman and Company, San Franscisco, 1960.

Davson, H. : *A Text Book of General Physiology,* Churchill, London, 1970.

Dickens, Randle and Whelan : *Carbohydrate-Metabolism and its Disorders,* Academic Press, New York, 1968.

Dickerson and Geis : *The Structure and Action of Proteins,* Academic Press, New York, 1973.

Eccles, J.C. : *The Physiology of Synapses,* Springer, Berlin, 1968.

Ernster and Drahota : *Mitochondrial Structure and Function,* Academic Press, New York, 1969.

Filley, G.F. : *Acid-Base and Gas Regulation,* Lea & Febiger, New York, 1971.

Florey, E. : *An Introduction to General and Comparative Animal,* Oxford University Press, New York, 1989.

Florkin and Stotz : *Comprehensive Biochemistry,* Elsevier, London, 1968.

Gene and Reynolds : *Water-soluble Vitamins,* John Wiley, London, 1963.

Gergely, J. : *Biochemistry of Muscle Contraction,* Little Brown & Company, Boston, 1964.

Goldberger, : *Water, Electrolyte, and Acid-Base Syndrome,* Lea & Febiger, New York, 1975.

Goodwin : *The Metabolic Roles of Citrate,* Academic Press, New York, 1970.

Gorbman, A. and Bern, H.A. : *A Text Book of Comparative Endocrinology,* John Wiley and Sons, New York, 1962.

Greenberg, Rodwell : *Amino Acid Metabolism,* Cambridge University Press, Cambridge, 1964.

Greenberg, Rodwell : *Carbon Catabolism of Amino Acids,* Academic Press, New York, 1969.

Gyorgy, Pearson : *The Vitamins,* Academic Press, New York, 1967.

Haldane, J.S. : *Respiration,* Yale University Press, New Haven, 1922.

Haldane, J.S. and Priestly, J.G. : *Respiration,* Oxford University Press, London, 1935.

Harrington, J.T. : *Clinimal Disorders of Urine,* Routledge, London 1973.

Harris, Loraine and Wool : *Vitamins and Hormones,* Academic Press, New York, 1967.

Harvey, Williams : *On the Motion of the Heard and Blood in Animals,* Cambrigde University Press, London, 1628.

Hoschemeyer and Hoschemeyer : *Proteins : A Guide to Physiology and Biochemistry,* John Wiley, London, 1991.

Huxley, H.E. : *The Mechanism of Muscular Conduction,* Spring Harbor, Harbor, 1972.

Jacobs and Wonvood : *Iron in Biochemistry and Medicine,* Academic Press, New York, 1968.

Jencks, : *Catalysis in Chemistry and Enzymology,* McGraw Hill, New York, 1961.

Johnson, A.R. : *Biochemistry and Methodology of Human* , John Wiley, London, 1971.

Katz, B. : *How Cells Communicate?*, W.H. Freeman & Co., California, 1661.

—— : *Nerve Muscle and Synapse,* McGraw Hill, New York, 1966.

Klahr, S. and Slatoposky E. : *Renal Regulation of Sodium Excretion,* Oxford University Press, London, 1973.

Koshland and Neet : *The Catalytic and Regulatory Properties of Enzymes,* Academic Press, New York, 1972.

Lehninger : *The Mitochondrion: Molecular Basis of Structure and Function,* MacMillan, London, 1966.

Lotspeick, W.D. : *Metabolic Aspects of Renal Function,* Thomas Publisher, New York, 1959.

Maxwell, M.H. and Kleeman C.R. : *Elements of Human Body,* McGraw Hill, New York, 1972.

McCance and Widdowson : *The Composition of Food,* Her Majesty's Office, London, 1960.

Meister : *Biochemistry of the Amino Acids,* Academic Press, New York, 1965.

Merler, E. : *Immunoglobulins : Biological Aspects and Clinical Uses,* Natural Academy of Sciences, Washington, 1970.

Openheimer, J.H. and Others : *Nuclear Receptors and the Initiation of Thyroid Jormone Action,* Little Brown and Company, Boston, 1976.

Prosser, Brown, : *Comparative Animal Physiology,* Saunder, Philadelphia, 1961.

Quirk, R. P. : *Chemistry of Muscular Contraction,* Academic Press, New York, 1970.

Ramot, B. : *Red Cell Structure and Metabolism,* Academic Press, New York, 1971.

Schmidt, Nelson K. : *Animal Physiology,* Prentice Hall, New Jersey, 1970.

Sela, M. : *New Perspectives in Biology,* American Elsevier, New York, 1963.

Shearman, R.P. : *Human Reproductive Physiology,* Blackwell, New York, 1972.

Shields, J.W. : *The Trophic Functions of Lymphoid Elements,* Spring-field, New York, 1972.

Shreeve, W.W. : *Physiological Chemistry of Carbohydrates in Mammals,* Saunders, New York, 1974.

Tullts, L.P. : *Blood Cells and Plasma Proteins : their State in Nature,* Academic Press, New York, 1953.

Tuttle, W.W. and Schottelius B.A. : *A Textbook of Physiology,* Mosby, Saint Louis, 1988.

Umland, J. B. : *Textbook of Physiology and Biochemistry,* West Pub., Co., London, 1972.

Underwood, E.J. : *Trace Elements in Human and Animal Nutrition,* Academic Press, New York, 1971.

Vender, A.J., Sherman J.H. and Luciano D.S. : *The Mechanisms of Body Function,* Tata McGraw, New York, 1975.

Wakil and Barnes : *Fatty Acid Metabolism,* Oxford University Press, London, 1971.

Walls, G. : *General Endocrinology,* WB Saunders and Co., Philadelphia, 1974.

West, E. S. and Others : *Text Book of Biochemistry,* MacMillan, London,1966.

Whelan : *Control of Glycogen Metabolism,* Academic Press, New York, 1968.

Williams, C.A. and Chase, M.W. : *Methods of Animal Physiology,* Academic Press, New York, 1968.

Williams, S.R. : *Animal Physiology,* MacMillan, London, 1973.

Yapp, W.B. : *An Introduction to Animal Physiology,* Clarendon Press, New York, 1960.

Zhukov, M. F. : *Organic Chemistry of Biological Compounds,* Englewood Cliffs, Prentice Hall, 1971.

Zumdahl, S. S. : *An Introduction to General and Comparative Physiology,* Oxford University Press, New York, 1981.

